is my child next?

THE ALEXA BROWN STORY

Jonathan Walsh

Copyright © 2020 by by Walsh Innovations. All rights reserved.

Walsh Innovations
6838 Mayapple Circle
Solon, OH 44139

This book or any portion thereof may not be reproduced or used in any manner whatsoever without the express written permission of the publisher except for the use of brief quotations in a scholarly work or book review. For permissions or further information contact Braughler Books LLC at:

   info@braughlerbooks.com

The views and opinions expressed in this work are those of the author and do not necessarily reflect the views and opinions of Braughler Books LLC.

Cover photo: Wendy Brown
Back cover photo of monument: Bev Henson

Printed in the United States of America
Published by Braughler Books LLC., Springboro, Ohio

First printing, 2020

ISBN: 978-1-970063-77-6 paperback
ISBN: 978-1-970063-67-7 hardcover
ISBN: 978-1-970063-60-8 ebook

Library of Congress Control Number: 2020905796

Ordering information: Special discounts are available on quantity purchases by bookstores, corporations, associations, and others. For details, contact the publisher at:

   sales@braughlerbooks.com

   or at 937-58-BOOKS

For questions or comments about this book, please write to:
   info@braughlerbooks.com

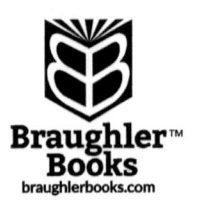

Braughler™ Books
braughlerbooks.com

"Alexa's name and the heart I scribed in the sand along with the portion of ashes we all spread are now fully committed to the ocean. High tide last night washed away one half and high tide today cared for the balance this morning. As she did in her struggle in life, she would not give up her name or her heart, even to the ocean until the last moment."

Warren in Ohio
On CaringBridge.com

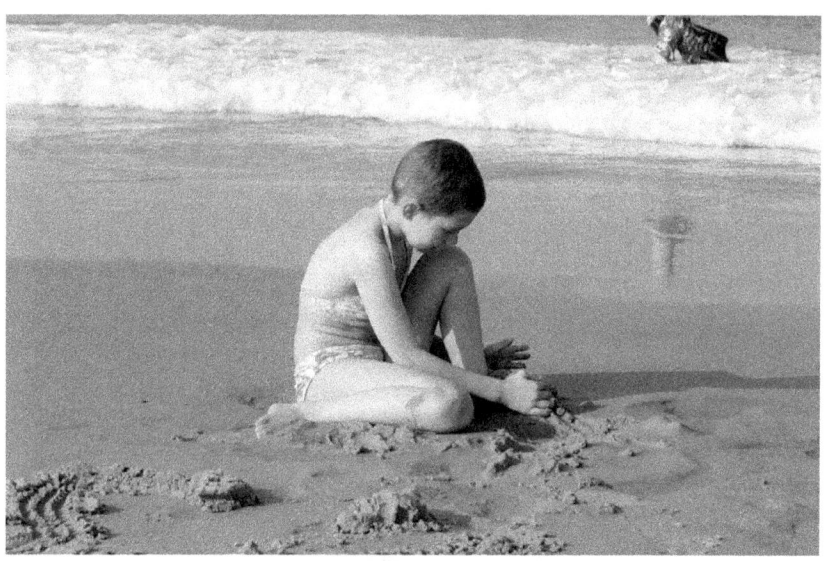

Alexa Brown on "Her Beach"

I have true admiration and sincere respect for the families involved in this book. I dedicate my writing to them, their strength, their courage, their struggle, and their healing.

Thank you to the communities that have given their time, talents, and love to all of these families when they needed it the most. Your dedication to those who've been hurt is a tremendous inspiration.

I would like to thank all of my family members for their love, support, and help with this book. You have been there with me through it all. I am deeply grateful for you and for God allowing me to be a part of your lives.

chapter 1

Wendy Brown handed out tiny glass containers that held the ashes of her little girl, Alexa Brown. These were the remains of Alexa's lost battle on earth, but ultimate victory in Heaven. Everyone, wearing Alexa's favorite color purple, stood on the clean sand as a gentle breeze swept across the lightly crashing waves nearby. About a dozen people were there to see the final, physical step of Alexa's journey.

Each person received a small bottle about the size of a thimble. Each bottle had a little cork cap. With that breeze flowing across the same beach where the Brown family vacationed each year, Wendy gave the blessing. Wendy's frail but determined voice was coming from a mother who saw the best of Alexa and the worst that life can bring. As she spoke, the sand became dotted with tears from everyone in attendance. "We have entrusted our beloved daughter, and sister, cousin and friend Alexa to God's mercy and we now commit her body to this beach, 'Alexa's Beach.'"

Each family member and friend opened his or her bottle, paused a moment, turned it upside down, and allowed Alexa to return to the place where she always wanted to be…her beach. The ashes floated onto the sand. Some covered the engraved heart and Alexa's name that her father, Warren Brown, had etched with a shovel into the beach. Some of Alexa flittered into the water. The waves crashed a bit harder enveloping the remains and claiming them for the ocean. The breeze picked up as if it knew to help carry Alexa. Just enough of her, though, knew to find its way to the feet of her parents.

As heads hung and tears flowed down the very cheeks that Alexa would kiss on a regular basis, Wendy uttered the final words. "Earth to earth. Ashes to ashes. Dust to dust."

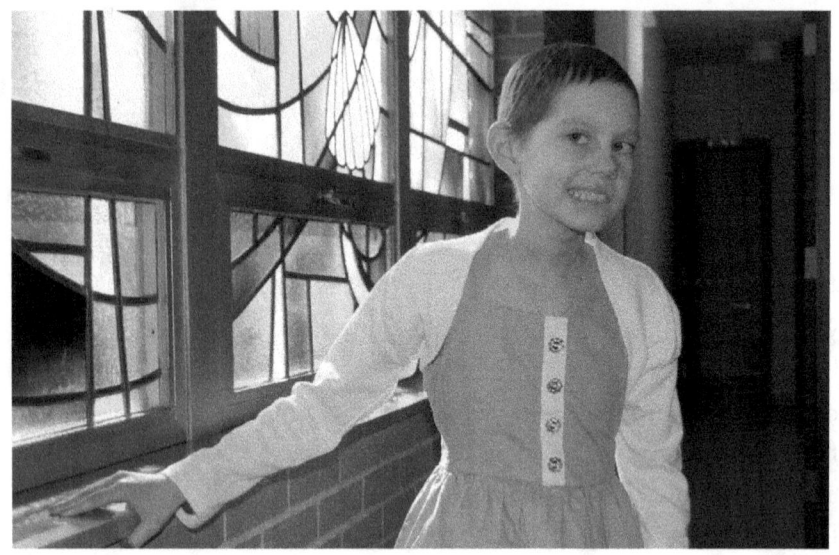

Alexa Brown

"What Cancer Cannot Do

It cannot cripple your love, it cannot shatter hope, it cannot corrode faith, it cannot destroy peace, it cannot kill friendship, it cannot suppress memories, it cannot silence courage, it cannot invade the soul, it cannot steal eternal life, it cannot conquer the spirit!!

I saw this, and I thought of you, Alexa. You have proven this to be true with your strength and your endless courage. Your spirits are always up higher than anyone could ever ask of you, and I know that you have not lost hope or faith in God that you will overcome this. Not a single day goes by that I am not inspired by your EXTRAORDINARY strength and courage. This is scary from the outside, yet you hold up stronger than most people around you. You are such a fighter, and that is why I have hope and faith that you will beat this."

Brandi from Ohio
On CaringBridge.com

chapter 2

The headline read, "County to Look Into 8 to 9 Cases of Children With Cancer." The cases were occurring in the same small area. The four-inch article got lost amidst the newsprint columns. My news director Mitch Jacob told me, "If this is true, this is one hell of a story."

With that, I was handed the newspaper and assigned to cover the story. He wanted it on air for the 6pm news. I was a television news anchor and investigative reporter in Toledo, OH. My name is Jonathan Walsh.

The breaking story I was about to uncover is mind-boggling. But in the moment, I was feeling rushed…pushed by my news director. "Do we really have to cover this for tonight?" I remember asking my boss. I was a bit uneasy with the sudden urgency.

I had no sooner taken my coat off, slumped it over my chair, and cleared the pile of papers from my keyboard when I was handed this story. It's something I've come to accept as a reporter. You go where the story is no matter what the time, or what the day. It's uncanny how, in the beginning, I felt "burdened" with this assignment. After just a few hours into it, however, I became impassioned by it. And the urgency my news director felt that morning is now my urgency to let the public know just how important this issue is.

Through all of this, I learned about children fighting for their lives, parents fighting for answers, and the residents of Ohio fighting the fear that any innocent child could contract the deadly disease. Parents always questioned, "Is my child next?"

Unfortunately, a diagnosis of cancer is all too common these days. But I always pictured the victims of this disease to be older adults who smoked all their lives, ate too much processed food, or spent too many hours in the tanning bed. I never—until now—pictured a five-year-old boy on his bike, a thirteen-year-old girl with freckles, or a seven-year-old turning cartwheels through her front yard.

An hour after reading the headline, my photographer Jeff Feasel and I were driving into that mostly rural northwest Ohio area. Beside the town park's water slide, there was a tall water tower that proudly displayed the name "Clyde." It's a place now in the middle of a mystery that, even to this day, has given people living there sleepless nights and untold sorrow.

The quaint and picturesque park was filled with volleyball courts, playground equipment and soccer fields. There was little action, though, until we spotted dirt clouds being kicked up by a girls' softball team running drills. We noticed a few adults sitting on the bleachers. They looked to be parents and grandparents planted on the dull silver slabs. "Grab the camera and I'll grab the mic," I told my photog. "Start taking shots of the practice and I'll try to find someone who has heard about this."

Scanning the faces of the spectators was difficult since they were all pretty much ignoring me. They were, however, starting to whisper to each other about the news van with the large WTOL logo. I turned toward the field and watched a group of tween girls with mitts on their hands, hair pulled back or in braids, intently listening to the shouts of their coach.

I started to wonder, "Are any of these girls part of these 8 or 9 cases? Do they know anyone who is? What about the coach? Does she know anything?"

Imagine me, a perfect stranger to these young girls, wondering if any of them were affected. I didn't even know about this town 24 hours earlier. And then, as I stood in the midst of the community, I felt engulfed by an unusual state of concern.

Now imagine, for a moment, that you're not an "outsider looking in;" that you're a parent of one of these young girls, a parent of any young person in this area or, much worse, you're a parent of a child who has mysteriously contracted one of these deadly cancers. My job was to take the imagination out of the equation, to present the public with the facts, and to show the heart of this terrible scenario.

After watching a few throws to first base and the coach barking out game-like situations, I turned my head to Jeff who had moved the camera closer to the fence just outside the field of play. He set the camera to take shots of the "crowd" in the bleachers and all of a sudden, I heard, "Oh, no." Parents in the bleachers started to cover their faces and laugh knowing they could end up on the news.

At that point I noticed a woman who did not seem to mind the camera. She continued to watch the practice just ahead of her on the field. I took my mic, casually walked over to the bleachers, stood beside her and looked out onto the diamond.

"You got a daughter out there?" I asked while keeping my eyes on the field and not making eye contact with the woman.

"A granddaughter," she responded. "She's pretty good." The woman smiled as her elbows were resting on her knees and her sunglasses were covering a good portion of her face.

I smiled still looking at the team. I could see out of the corner of my eye that her head had turned to look at me. As my mic was hanging along my waistband, I also noticed her glance down to see the mic flag with our WTOL logo on it.

"You guys doing a story down here?" she asked. "These girls could use some coverage," she said with a smile.

"I bet they could," I replied with a smirk and my eyes still glued on the drills the girls were playing out. "But I'm actually here on a different story," I added as I took a seat in the stands.

"You know anything about a bunch of kids getting cancer down here?" I asked now looking into her sunglasses.

"Ooohhh," the grandma said turning her head, adjusting her position on the bleacher and fixing her sunglasses. "Yeah, I've heard about that."

"You know anyone who's in that group of 8 or 9 kids?" I asked.

"No, but I bet my granddaughter knows them," the older woman said as she pointed her index finger toward the field.

"Would you like to talk to us about that? We're trying to get people in the community to tell us how they feel," I explained as I held up the mic.

"Sure, but you probably should talk to the coach since she works with the kids here," the woman said.

As I interviewed the grandmother who I came to know as Betty Pocock, I could tell she did not know much about the cases. All I could gather was that she wanted more information from those who were investigating the outbreak of pediatric cancer.

"It could be in the air, something in the soil, something we're eating," Betty said in a way that sounded like she was thinking out loud. "I sure hope they figure it out."

After the brief interview, I needed to talk to the coach and maybe some of the kids, too. As it turned out, none of the children wanted to go on camera, but Coach Marilyn Lynch braved the mic.

"It's talked about quite a bit," Marilyn told us as the tape was rolling.

Apparently, it was such a huge topic in town, it was affecting her 12-year-old daughter, Kaitlyn, who also played on the team.

"She comes home from school wanting to know if it's in the water," explained Marilyn with a concerned look on her own face. "She's pretty scared," she told me looking back onto the field at her daughter who was taking a sip of water from her water bottle.

"I just know a lot of parents are really concerned and it would be helpful to get a little bit more information," Marilyn continued as she swung her head back toward the mic and looked at me.

I thanked Marilyn and Betty for their time and waved to the girls.

"Byeee," the girls said smiling back at me. All I could think about was how young and innocent they were. Kids just trying to be kids and have some fun, all the while knowing there was something definitely wrong in their community.

My photographer packed up the gear and slammed the back gate of the Jeep Liberty. He made his way to the car and asked, "Where to next?"

"We need more information," I told him while looking through my yellow legal pad of notes from different past stories I had done and trying to find a phone number I wrote down when we were back at the station.

"Here it is," I said finding the number to the Sandusky County Health Department. "I hope this guy is still in his office."

I flipped open the phone, started to dial and we began weaving through Clyde. It's a small community that has a hometown feel. For the most part, the homes were built decades ago but kept up nicely. We could see parents walking with their kids, children playing in their yards and laughing as they played tag, and an older couple sitting on their front porch enjoying a nice night. I noticed the quaint downtown filled with hair salons, a gas station, a couple of restaurants, and a park in the middle of them all. I remember thinking, this reminds me of my hometown.

All of these observations were made while we were trying to get back to Fremont. That is the county seat and home to the health department. My thoughts of home were interrupted by someone saying, "Hello?" on the other end of the phone. I paused a second to gather my focus. "Is Dave Pollick available?" I asked.

Dave Pollick was the Health Commissioner, a man who stands about 6'2" with a mix of grey and dark brown hair, glasses, and a monotone voice that you would guess would be that of a scientist.

The health department office was quite small with a few employees sitting behind large-walled cubicles where stacks upon stacks of case folders and papers were piled up. I remember thinking, 'How do they keep track of those folders?'

Dave ushered us into his office and we sat down to do the interview. We were in the month of May so it was a bit warmer outside and his office had a stale-air feel to it. Fortunately, the interview was not as stale.

He told us that since last fall he had been looking into the cases that span from Clyde to nearby Green Creek Township and Green Springs. Of the 8-9 cases, he told us he had put together seven complete histories of the young patients. Their files were then forwarded to a state epidemiologist. He explained that it was "a process" that could take quite some time to figure out if there was something actually causing the cancer. Little did we know just how right he would be.

"I wish I could give a quicker answer. I will say we will do everything in our power to get that info moved along as quickly as possible," said Dave.

As we headed back to the station, the only way I could look over the tape was to play it through the camera. So, I picked out the soundbites with that 25-pound camera digging into my lap.

I did not completely realize what I was getting myself into. It was the start of what has become a life-changing commitment to help not only these children in Northwest Ohio, but to help give a voice to those families who were not able to truly speak for themselves as they dealt with the nightmare that is childhood cancer.

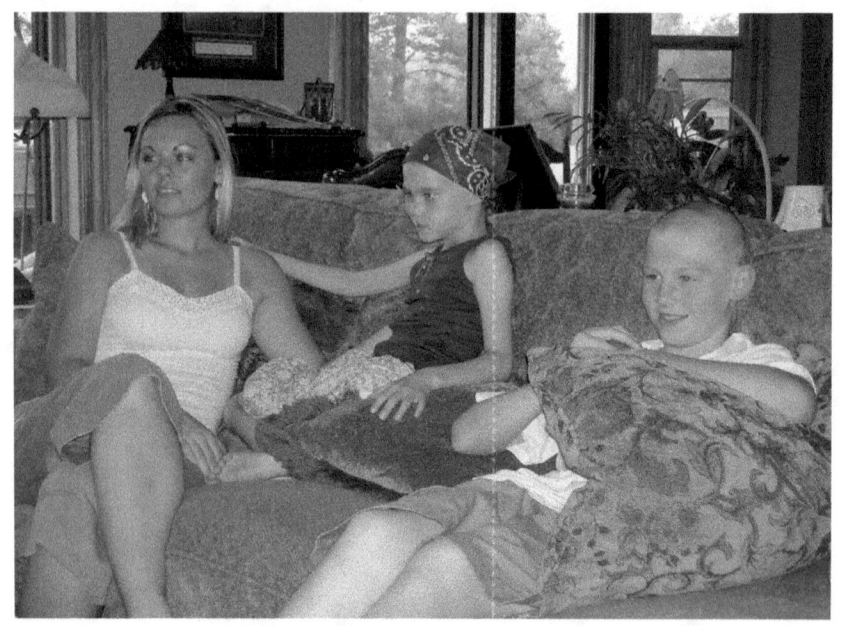

Amanda Brown, Alexa Brown, Ethan Brown

"Alexa, one more thing. I noticed that you've now had almost 50,000 visitors. You'll recall I was number 10,000. Well, I'm keeping my eye on the number. Maybe there are some of your friends and family out there that might want to join the challenge of becoming your 50,000th visitor. Lindsay? Alicia? Emily? Andrew? Sheryl? Ethan? Ronnie? Ray? Game on!"

Randy from Ohio
On CaringBridge.com

chapter 3

It was now two days after my first report. We had gotten a ton of attention from that story. On that afternoon, as I was coming into work, I was walking from the station's parking lot that is located on the banks of the Maumee River. I noticed a young girl probably 10 years-old or so fishing along the banks. She had on a pink coat, jeans, and a smile on her face as she stood by a man who I assumed was her dad. She had nothing to do with the cancer cluster, but it's children like her who've been affected.

As I stood there with my suit coat on a hanger in my hand and my black workbag slung over my shoulder, I could not help but think about my upcoming interview. It was the first of June in 2007 and it would turn out to be the first real day of my eye-opening experience involving this cancer cluster and, in general, children living with the disease.

All I could think about during my walk down the hall to my desk that day was getting on the phone before the interview and making sure 13-year-old Tyler Smith was well enough to talk with us. I tracked down her family after making calls and people in the community told me a few names of those who were in the thick of the mystery.

When I had talked to Tyler's mom and dad, Donna and Dave Hisey, they briefly described the brutal toll the radiation and chemo had taken as doctors tried to attack the leukemia surging through Tyler's little body.

I plopped my bag down on what many would describe as a messy desk that was full of videotapes, scripts and notes from previous reports, folders of special projects, and notable mementos of prior stories. I called my desk "organized confusion".

As I confirmed the interview, my news director made his way behind my corner desk and was pacing back and forth while I was on the phone.

"Is she okay?" he asked as I was literally hanging up the phone. I turned around in my swivel chair and saw his arms crossed and his right hand cupping his chin.

"We're heading to St. V's at four o'clock," I said.

"Good," he muttered as he turned quickly and walked back to his office.

I got up to go to our normal, daily newsroom 3:30pm meeting. Our news meeting area consisted of a converted cubicle about 10' x 12' with really dirty carpet and a large, rectangular table that had probably been recycled from a former conference room. Producers, reporters, anchors and managers all gathered around with sheets of paper sitting in front of every mismatched chair that lined the table. The papers outlined the stories of the day and who was covering what.

I got to the meeting a couple minutes later than everyone else because of my phone call to the Hiseys. All the good chairs were taken so I walked up to the maroon, stained seat that literally once had wheels but were now mysteriously absent. The left armrest was missing, too.

As I stared at the assignments for the day, each story had a title and brief description about what the report was covering. I then noticed my name on the list. I panned to the left to see the words "Cancer Cluster." I thought it was a bit premature to call it a "cluster" at this point since health leaders were just getting started in the study, but I knew the title was probably inspired by my news director. So, I just made a mental note instead of a vocal one.

The meeting adjourned and I walked back to my desk. My photographer emerged from a video editing bay.

"What's shakin' tonight?" he asked.

"We're heading to St. V's soon, so are you packed up and ready to roll?" I asked him.

"Give me five minutes and meet me out front," he said as he turned to go get his gear.

Amid all the papers and notes, sat that little newspaper article on my desk. I picked it up, looked at it, and thought "cancer cluster?" Maybe that title will fit by the time I learn more.

It took all of four minutes to get to the children's hospital at St. V's. It is literally just up the street from our station. I had never been in the children's area before and I did not know what to expect.

I waited for the hospital communications rep to meet us in the lobby so she could escort us to Tyler's room. It was hard to miss the big, bronze statue of St. Marguerite d'Youville standing right near the welcome desk. She helped form the Grey Nuns in Canada which was a group dedicated to charity work. Their tireless efforts included helping orphaned and abandoned children. Marguerite herself was a mother of two boys, but she had also suffered terrible loss. Four of her six children died at a very young age. How fitting it was that as I stared at the beautiful statue, now many decades later, she was still watching over children. Her Grey Nuns group helped start what is now known as St. Vincent Mercy Medical Center in Toledo, OH. Tyler was in the children's hospital at St. V's.

"This one's kind of a mystery, I hear," said the hospital communications representative as she approached me. Still with my eyes locked on that statue, I managed to softly reply, "That's for sure."

We started walking and she was making conversation as we entered the elevator. I'm not entirely sure what she was saying as my mind was still preoccupied thinking of Marguerite's story of her unhealthy kids. I looked back at the statue one last time and blurted out, "Yeah, they're looking into it." Just as I said that, I made room on the elevator for my photographer, his tripod, and single stand-light.

After a short ride, the elevator doors re-opened. There was an uncanny silence mixed with bright, warm, childlike colors on the walls. It was a strange combination…silence and youth.

There were pictures on the walls that appeared to be made by children. Many filled with bright blue skies and yellow suns…a stark contrast to what they were going through during their time at the hospital. I assumed the patients and their family members spent an awful lot of time there.

As the three of us turned a corner, I noticed a child in a wheelchair sitting in a waiting area watching a cartoon. No one was around her. Mom and Dad were probably talking with the nurse about what was to come that day. The little girl had an IV hanging from a cold, metal pole standing high above her chair. The pole was another glowing contrast to the brilliant paint, pictures, and lively children's TV show that built the atmosphere of the waiting area.

While we walked the maze of hallways, I saw more children. Some were walking with a limp. Others were being wheeled in a bed with nurses and concerned parents at their sides. I saw one child walking toward me with a white, oversized gauze bandage around his head and he was toting the all-too-common IV pole on wheels. The one thing that struck me in that brief couple of seconds was his size. With sick kids, there is no normal height and weight, no healthy glowing skin that children often have, no sense of age because their bodies have endured so much.

My eyes followed the boy as he opened the waiting room door. I saw several parents who looked more tired than anyone should. They were sitting in chairs lining the walls, watching their little ones trying to play with toys left in the room, and passing the time between treatments.

All of the images hit me, but I kept walking, not really hearing the continued small talk of the communications rep until she stopped in front of Tyler's hospital room door.

"She has just gotten a treatment today, but she's feeling pretty good," the rep informed me. "I do have to warn you. I'm not sure if her parents told you, but Tyler is losing her hair so don't be surprised to see that," she added.

"No problem," I said as she opened the door.

Right away I saw Dave and Donna Hisey sitting in chairs just off to the left side of Tyler's bed. Donna's eyes looked tired and Dave appeared to be in a bit of a daze as they shook my hand.

Donna was a beautiful woman with shoulder-length hair. She was wearing a sweatshirt and jeans…comfort clothing that was all-too-necessary when someone spends night after night alongside a sick loved one. I could tell her attractive face was hidden a bit by the wear-and-tear of the unexpected battle lines of pediatric cancer. Dave was a thin man with a goatee and a short haircut. As he stood, we could look each other in the eyes. What I saw was a worried, weary father who was still putting up a strong front so his family couldn't see his overall pain.

"Nice to meet you," I said. Donna's grip was weak.

"I wish it were under different circumstances," I added.

"We do, too," said Donna as her slumbered eyes look over to her first-born child lying in the bed.

I turned to see the 13-year-old. Her eyes were red. Her hair was virtually non-existent. Her body was covered with a hospital gown. I thought to myself, "No child should look like that."

Tyler was paying attention to her two younger siblings who were sitting at the foot of the bed. They were laughing and talking about something. I was not paying attention to their specific conversation, but rather their interaction. Instead of being outside in their front yard, this family had playtime in a place where play is used as a distraction from a harsh reality.

"And you must be Tyler," I said with a smile holding out my hand to shake hers.

"Yup," she said with a smile. "Nice to meet you," she told me. The kids turned their attention to us.

"These must be your brother and sister?" I asked.

"Yeah, that's Tanner and that's Sierra," Tyler told me, pointing out the healthy children of the family. Tanner is a few years younger than Tyler with a thin face, light brown hair and a normal-looking build. Sierra is a couple of years younger than Tanner with the cutest face and a full head of beautiful hair—something I bet Tyler would love to have.

"Hi, guys. Looks like you are having fun," I said to the younger siblings, knowing none of this was fun for anyone.

"We try," said Tanner as he hopped off the bed pulling Sierra with him.

"How are you feeling?" I asked turning my attention back to the near-bald young lady propped up by pillows in the bed.

"Pretty good. I've been here a while now, but we make the best of it," she said with a smile. She then took off her glasses and rubbed her already bloodshot eyes. She got drops placed into her eyes every once in a while, during the day to help offset some of the side effects of treatment.

It has not been an easy life for Tyler. Her father passed away when she was just three years old and now, she has been diagnosed with cancer.

Dave is her stepfather but one who has been there most of her life. "How can this be happening?" Dave asked me. He described the overnight stays that were typically done by Donna while he took care of Tanner and Sierra. "They miss their mom and they miss their sister," he told us, talking about the younger kids.

"It hurts. Really hurts," said Donna with tears welling up in her eyes. She told us that before all the chemo treatments and even before the diagnosis, the family knew of other children in the community who had been struck by cancer, including a girl Tyler's age.

"I was in a women's group and I made a supper for the mother of one of the kids with cancer and I was never thinking we would ever go through anything like this ourselves," Donna admitted in a frail voice.

"When it happens to you, you understand exactly what they were going through," Dave said as he reached over to grasp his wife's hand.

"I tested the pond water. I tested the well water. I tested for radon," Dave said as he described his fruitless search for answers. "Not one of those tests came back abnormal."

Tyler told us, "I was really scared because I've never gone through anything like it." She was describing hearing the words, "Tyler, you have cancer."

Donna, Dave and Tyler also talked about the grueling schedule getting her to Toledo for weeks on end. It is about an hour-long drive from their home near Clyde to the hospital. Add to that work, kids, and school and you can see why Donna and Dave showed signs of extreme fatigue.

I told them about my visit with the Sandusky Health Department and how the state was getting involved with the investigation. The Hiseys were all too familiar with what was going on in their community.

"I prayed really hard that Tyler would be the last child in Clyde that would have cancer, but two months later, another person from our church…their child had it and we know her very well," Donna said with the same watery-eyed look that I saw when we first started the interview.

"You worry about your other kids," Dave jumped in. "Are they going to get something?" he asked looking over at Tanner and Sierra. Little did he know how prevalent that question would soon be for his once-healthy family.

That night, as I stood in front of the hospital waiting for the on-air coverage to begin, I wondered about what it must be like for the parents of these kids. What about the other families in the community who have no idea what is happening in their hometown?

I did my introduction to the taped piece and, as the story ended, I was live again to finish my report.

"This family says the community of Clyde has been extremely supportive by holding fundraisers, sending cards, and saying prayers," I reported staring into the camera with the children's hospital lit up behind me in the night sky. "But even with that support, these cancer cases have thrown questions into their lives. Should they move from the area to keep their other kids safe? Are they going to have to worry about every little cold thinking is this the start of cancer? Is life ever going to be the same? Reporting live in north Toledo, I'm Jonathan Walsh…News 11."

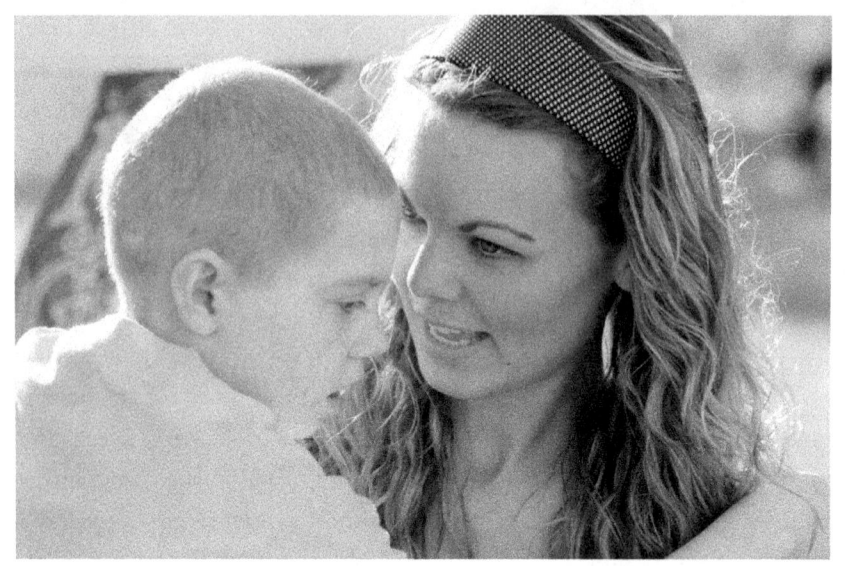

Alexa Brown, Amanda Brown

"Alexa, I know you don't know me but....

I just got your address from Aunt Cheryl and wanted to let you know that you are faithfully in our thoughts and prayers!!! Praying you will feel up to going home ASAP!!

I have often prayed that I would gladly take your place if only the Lord would allow me. Just know you are loved. I have also had cancer twice in the last 4 yrs. and Jesus has faithfully been with us each step of the way!

Again, we love you!!"

Darlene from New Jersey
On CaringBridge.com

chapter 4

As my investigation into these cancer cases grew deeper, I was meeting with families who have had their lives turned upside down now that their children were part of this exclusive and never-desirable group of kids. Jessica and Jeremy Ferkel had one of those families.

As I pulled up to the Ferkel's home in rural Riley Township, I noticed the modest, ranch-style house and the older cars in the driveway. It struck me that none of these families in this study were more than middle class. In fact, many were just barely getting by. Paycheck to paycheck was the reality they faced. Many times, mom and dad were getting plenty of help from their moms and dads. The Ferkels were no exception.

I was introduced to the Ferkels and their son, Chase Berger, through Jane Hemmer. Jane was an attractive grandma who stood no taller than 5'2" but was full of chutzpa. She knew what had happened to her grandson was not right and she was ready to tell the world about it.

I stepped out of our Jeep Liberty with the blazing decals of WTOL News 11 on the sides, walked to the back and told my photographer, "I'm not sure what kind of shape this kid is in. So, just be ready for anything."

Jane was married to Russell Fritz. Russell was a handsome older man with grey hair but not old-looking. He was in good shape with a bit of a shadow on his face from a few days without a shave. He greeted us as we walked along the gravel driveway. "Can I give you a hand with that?" Russell asked, pointing to the equipment in our hands.

"Oh, no. That's all right. I have to do something more than just carry a pen," I replied with a smile.

Russell kindly laughed and said, "I'm Russ, Chase's grandpa. We appreciate you coming out to talk to us. This problem needs to see the light of day."

I told him with the smile still on my face, "It needs a bigger spotlight than the sun, but we'll do the best we can."

As I walked in, the door creaked and opened to a house with furniture that appeared to be 20 years old. Nicely decorated, but smaller and a bit dated.

"I'm Jessica," said Chase's mom standing up from the kitchen table. She was a young mom in her 20's with a pretty face that showed the telltale signs of stress. She was a bit shy but managed a grin as she extended her hand for a friendly shake.

"I'm Jonathan. Great to meet you," I said taking her hand into mine and looking into her tired eyes. "Jane tells me it's been a rough few months for you guys. You're not alone, unfortunately," I added.

"It has been rough for us," she said with a sigh but managing a smile. "My husband is still at work but he should be here any moment now," she explained. Just then, a little guy walked into the room wearing sunglasses so dark you could not see his eyes. "Oh," Jessica said taking notice of the little man. "And this is Chase."

Chase was 5 years old with a buzz haircut. He was a skinny kid whose shirt hung loosely on his frail frame. He was a bit pale and small for his age, but appeared to be full of energy.

"Well, hello there, big man," I said to him while bending down to shake his hand.

He barely got out a "hi" before lightly shaking my hand then turning to his mom for a hug. He was a little shy and/or embarrassed. I couldn't figure it out just yet.

As we set up the light and the camera, I sat at the table across from Jessica. Jane and Russ were in the room, too. As I turned to get comfortable in my chair, I saw Jane facing Russ rubbing his arms. Russ had a can't-believe-my-child-and-grandchild-are-in-this-situation look on his face as his eyes pointed to the ground. Jane tried to comfort him.

"I have been talking to others involved with this study," I told

Jessica, who was sitting with her hands folded, elbows on the table, trying to be brave.

"I've wondered how they are dealing with all of this, too," she said staring at me. "You know there've been times when I've had to hold Chase's head out of the toilet because he's so lifeless and laying on the bathroom floor," she added with her eyes welling up.

"I can't even imagine what you've already been through," I said.

During our conversation, I told her I wanted to understand as much as a person who is not directly in the study can understand.

"You tell me as much as you want," I said tapping her hand. "And we'll let people know what's happening," I added. No sooner did my words end then Jeremy Ferkel walked through the back door attached to the kitchen.

"Sorry, I'm late," said Jeremy shaking my hand. Jeremy was a young man who was handsome in his own right. He was a taller guy with a baby face and a look as rundown as his wife's appearance revealed.

As the two parents sat at the table and poured their hearts out about their little boy, I could tell immediately they were very involved in their son's life. There was a hint of a previous divorce and past relationships from their conversations, but from the various last names involved coming into the interview, I had a feeling there would be some of that. However, they genuinely seemed to like each other and wanted nothing more than to help make Chase feel that he was just like everyone else. It was not an easy goal considering the little guy's cancer attacked a section of his face near his right eye.

His parents told me Chase had to wear sunglasses all the time because light could be painful. His eye was constantly red and it bothered him immensely.

"Between me and him, we used to be really close," said Jessica. "Now it's 'I hate you! I don't like you!' He slaps me. He kicks me," she added with more tears ready to stream down her young, worried face.

Jeremy told me that was one of the most difficult aspects of this disease. Other than the physical pain that he saw his son going through on a daily basis, Jeremy said Chase had become a completely different boy since the diagnosis in January of 2006. Jeremy knew this was just the beginning.

"He's got to deal with this for his whole life," he told me with a strain in his voice.

The interview lasted about 20 minutes and then Chase decided to take his glasses off. He revealed a swollen eye that had streaks of red racing through the white. It was as bloodshot of an eye that I had ever seen. The light hurt him so badly he could not look up at me. He tried. It just did not happen.

"We need to know what's going on here," said Jane during our talk. "There's just too many cancer cases in this town. It's unbelievable," she added with the same bewildered look as the rest of her family had ever since we walked through the door.

"That's the frustrating thing," Russ blurted out. "It's just all these little kids and they haven't had a chance at life, you know? That's what hurts the most," he finished with a furrowed brow and his hand stroking his facial scruff.

Chase did not say much to us during the interview but he was very interested in showing us his bedroom full of racing memorabilia. He led us to his room down the hall. In the small 10' x 10' bedroom, there was racing legend Jeff Gordon stuff everywhere with a bunch of John Deere tractor items, too.

While we were enjoying the tour of his room, he gradually became a little more comfortable with us. We showed interest in the things he liked. Without any cue from us or his parents, Chase pulled up his shirt and revealed his IV port.

"This is where I get my medicine," he said pointing to the scar tissue and the tiny yellow-looking tube that hung from his chest.

I had never seen a port before and here was one about two feet from my eyes on the skinniest, palest, littlest chest. How real was that? A five-year-old so familiar with this medical treatment that he could teach me a thing or two about what life can be like.

"You are brave, my man," I told Chase trying to keep him comfortable even though it was probably me who needed a moment to gather myself.

"Yeah," he said as he put his shirt back down and headed back out of the room.

As we wrapped up the shoot, we got some great pictures of Chase riding his bike like a "normal" kid his age. We rattled off more video of him hugging his mom and grandparents who more than likely felt that port poking through his thin t-shirt.

During that evening's 11pm newscast, I stood in the studio watching the taped report I had just put together and then delivered the close to the story.

"Chase's family tells News 11 he still has bad cells in him and even when it looks like their all gone, with this type of cancer, 90% of the time it comes back and it can show up in another place in his body."

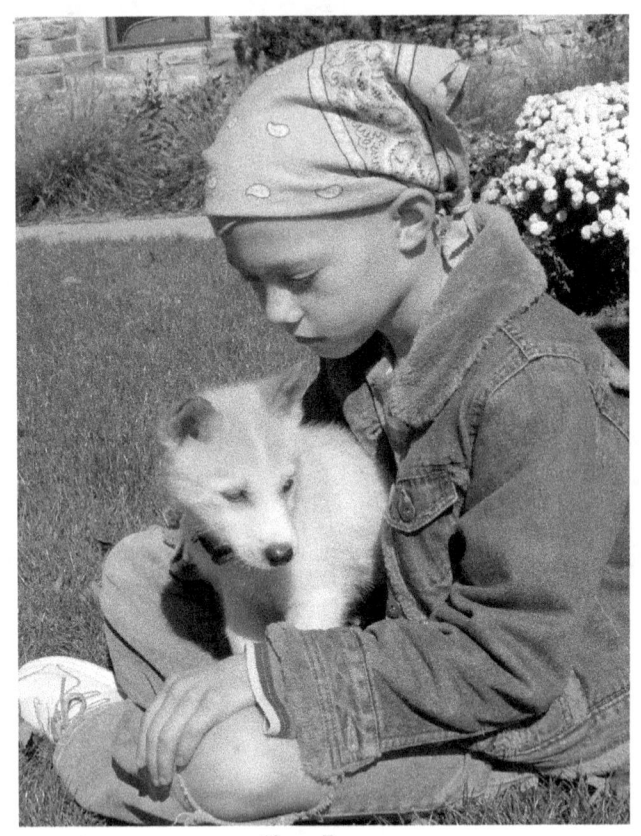

Alexa Brown

"Hi Alexa!

Thanks for the nice card you sent us. We are keeping up with your news on this great website and think of you a lot! It's like the story of Supergirl—you are super!

Lots of love,

Ronnie, Doug and Diana from New Jersey"
On CaringBridge.com

chapter 5

A few weeks after our story with Chase and his family, I found myself on a short drive from the hospital to work. My mind was racing. I was motivated even more to keep on top of this medical mystery that stole childhoods one cancer cell at a time. All because of a visit I paid Tyler Smith minutes before.

My wife and I had put together a get-well-soon bag for hospital-ridden Tyler. I had remembered her mom saying Tyler liked scrapbooking. My wife has a creative mind, has a great way with pictures, and enjoys the hobby as well. She gathered up some paper and stickers for me to take to Tyler in the hospital.

St. V's was just a few blocks from the station, so before I went into work, I stopped by the children's section of the hospital. I will never forget the visit.

I wanted to surprise Tyler and Donna, so I just made my way up to the nurse's station and asked to see Tyler. The nurse informed me Tyler had taken a turn for the worse and was now in the ICU. Donna was by her side.

At first, I thought I should just leave, but then theorized that maybe I could bring some cheer to the family with a quick 'hello.'

As I was led up to Tyler's ICU room, the space was so quiet I could not hear a thing. It was hard to believe, but the silence was even more deafening than the other portions of the children's treatment area.

After a long walk down a bare hallway, I passed the nurse's station where even their conversation seemed hushed. I came to Tyler's door. "Wait here," said the nurse wearing brightly colored scrubs probably in an effort to keep things as cheery as possible in a place where many children have spent their final days.

Donna emerged from the room. Her face was clearly worn, skin pale, and shoulders hunched as if she had just spent the night sleeping on one of those foldout beds that turn into an uncomfortable chair.

She tried to manage a smile but the look of concern was deep in her eyes. Her exhausted body language spoke volumes about just how serious this turn in health had become.

I was stunned. I was standing there with a white, plastic grocery bag filled with the fun scrapbooking supplies. However, at that moment when I fully took in Donna's despair, I completely doubted any plan I had.

"Hi," I said with pursed lips and a half-smile as if I was really saying, "I know this completely and utterly sucks and I am so sorry for what you're going through." I gave her a hug, but her embrace was weak.

"How's she doing?" I asked Donna who was now looking at the ground and seemed in a daze. Who could blame her?

"She's doing all right," she told me very unconvincingly as her brown hair hung lifelessly now over her face. "She's had a rough couple of days and they're hoping this is the worst of it before she bounces back." Tears started to build in her eyes.

"I'm so sorry, Donna," I told her, extending my hand and touching her cold arm. She nodded.

There was silence…the kind that probably lasted a couple of seconds but felt like an eternity as we both stood there wondering what else there was to say. I thought about the last time I saw Tyler. She was sitting up, playing games with her siblings, and joking with me as I was talking into the video camera describing what our viewers will see during her story. Other than her visibly balding head, you would not have known this kid was in the battle of her life. Now that had never been truer.

"I remember you telling me how much Tyler liked scrapbooking," I finally said to break the dead, still air. The crinkling sound from the plastic bag helped continue the noise as I opened the bag to show Donna what I brought. "I thought she could break up the routine in her room with these and a few of her pictures, but I had no idea she was up here now," I said, referring to the ICU.

Donna glanced into my eyes with a blank stare that told me too much was happening for her to comprehend. "Thank you, Jonathan," she said.

"I even brought some golf-themed stuff because I remember her saying how much she likes to golf," I said in a cheerier voice trying to put something positive out there in an otherwise dark atmosphere. It was not working.

"That's really nice of you," she told me as she took the bag and looked inside. "She really does like to golf," she added with a half-hearted smile.

"My wife found some other great supplies that she thought a teenage girl would enjoy," I said furthering the conversation.

Donna looked up at me, "Tell her thank you, too."

More silence took over the hallway. It engulfed us. I could not even hear the nurses who had since left the station and were walking into another room. I was so focused on what to say next, but nothing came out.

"Would you like to see her?" Donna asked. I did not know how to respond.

This situation was one of those private moments in a family's life and I did not want to intrude.

I kind of looked at her to see if she was serious. "Only if you think it's okay," I said in a concerned voice.

"Yeah. Come on in. But just to let you know she's sleeping and not looking all that well," Donna warned.

As she pushed open the oversized, cold, wooden door, it didn't make a sound. What were noticeable were the machines running in that dark ICU room.

I made sure to pay attention to where I was walking so as not to disturb anything. I strode past the corner of the hospital bed and there was Tyler. It was unlike anything I had ever seen before.

She slept but not in a calm way. Her body looked angry—battling this next stage of her cancer fight. She had on one of those thin blue hospital nightgowns, loosely placed on her ghostly skin. Who knows how many children had worn that particular gown before and that never made it through the treatment.

Tyler was also wrapped in what looked like a white canvas body suit almost like a cast that was attached to pumps.

I remember Donna tried to explain what treatment the doctors had now employed, but my mind was honed in on this young lady who in no way shape or form should be here. This scenario only played out with old people, those who had lived long lives and were trying to hold on for just a bit more time. This was no place for a child who had barely known anything past Barbie, sixth grade math, and that new awkward feeling of thinking a boy in her class was cute.

"Basically, they're hoping this pumping action will get some of the bad stuff out," Donna said in a whispered voice. To this day, I have no idea what that process was designed to do, but I can clearly recall watching Tyler's young, battered body clinging to life.

Even with my good intentions, I knew it was time for me to leave this mother with her first born. "I will be praying for you, Donna," I said.

"Thank you," she replied.

I left Donna that day with another new perspective; the slightest of insights into just what thousands of kids and their families have to deal with on any given day.

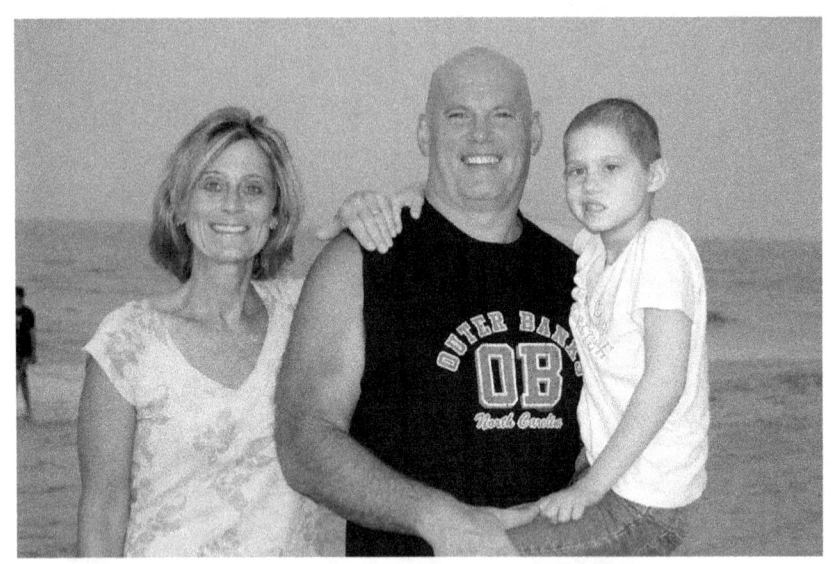

Wendy Brown, Warren Brown, Alexa Brown

"It is a sunny and dry day here in Rugby, England, quite unusual now, because although it is summer, we have had quite a bit of rain! I decided to come inside to check my emails and found my update from your site, so with bated breath I opened it, as it is normally later in the day that it is updated! I was so pleased to read that things are o.k. with you all, and I am sending my love and prayers across the sea to the U.S.A. You are an incredible family and my thoughts are with you."

Sharon Rugby from United Kingdom
On CaringBridge.com

chapter 6

"I wonder where we can set up," I told my photographer as we walked into an old, gray building.

There was a community room toward the back of the first floor where an event was taking place. Large tables set up in a row made it look more like a soup kitchen with old metal chairs dotting the sides. There was music playing and I noticed a café tucked away in the corner. It was more like a counter and a chalkboard menu than a real café, but the lounge chairs and couch made it feel more like a coffee shop that just happened to be attached to a soup kitchen.

"Why don't we just have them sit on the couch?" I mentioned to my photographer.

As he pulled out the long thin metal legs for the one and only light, we had in the back of our news truck, I looked around at the dark lobby. Plain walls, oversized chairs, and a dated coffee table made up the décor. With the bright light finally balanced on the tiny metal stand, I noticed a tall, thin, young woman walking with an older woman at her side.

My photographer started rolling. It was Shilah Donnersbach.

Shilah, at the age of 19, was the oldest victim in the cancer study at the time. She was a small-town girl who, with all her might, tried to be as stylish as she could. A nice pair of jeans and a thin, dressy shirt with sparkles. It hung on her tiny frame with noticeable bagginess. There was one more "accessory" Shilah did not want to have on: her leg brace.

Shilah limped with a noticeably thinner, right leg. The older woman bracing Shilah's stride was her mother, Trina Donnersbach. Trina's eyes looked as exhausted as she felt. She held onto Shilah's arm as they made their way through the lobby.

Trina wore a nice sweater and an older pair of jeans. She had the body language of a woman who had just gotten off first-shift and was in-between her next part-time job. It was a drained feeling this mother wore after having watched her daughter's body worn out by cancer.

"Hi, Trina? I'm Jonathan Walsh. Nice to finally meet you in person," I said with a smile as she walked by me to the couch.

I tracked Trina down through a number of channels in the community. The Sandusky Health Department would not release any names of patients involved in the cancer study. HIPAA laws did not allow that. So, I was forced to network and get bits and pieces of info about the victims from those in town who were "in the know."

"And you must be, Shilah," I said as the two women were adjusting themselves on the couch.

Shilah managed to produce a smile from her gaunt, freckly face. Her small glasses were tucked between the hairs in her auburn-colored wig. Chemo claimed her real hair, too.

As we eased into the interview, Shilah described the problems with her leg. "I lost all the strength in it because of it being so painful," she said. "I tried staying off of it," she added. The odd thing is, the cancer never was in her leg. She actually had a tumor the size of a grapefruit in her pelvic region. The cancer then spread and affected her leg.

"Doctors tell us now that if they do surgery at any point, they will cut my leg off," Shilah said as she cupped her tired leg with both hands surrounding the brace. I could tell she was uncomfortable.

All the while, Trina watched from her sad eyes…probably thinking, "How did we get here?" Is this really happening? Will my daughter survive?"

Trina jumped into the conversation. "I would hear her screaming at night," she told us. "Crying because of the pain," she added. This new world for her and her daughter took some time to sink in. "It was very difficult to even imagine," said Trina. "I mean, we've never had anyone in the family diagnosed with cancer," she said as her words trailed off and she looked down. It was as if she was going over the scenario in her head for the millionth time.

Shilah was already a lean girl to begin with, but the cancer had shed another 30 pounds from her skinny frame. Admittedly, at times, cancer had shed her will, too.

"You want to give up sometimes and I don't even want to do treatments any more. I just want to give up," she told us in a desperate voice. However, there was no way she could give up. Shilah was a mother to a one-and-a-half-year-old boy.

"If we don't move away and we do stay here in Clyde, I don't want my son to have the same problem," Shilah groaned. The struggle between familiarity and family roots versus common sense was a battle in her mind.

Trina's motherly heart ached for her daughter who was now a mommy herself. "It is very difficult because there's nothing I can do but be there with her, pray with her, hold her hand," Trina uttered in a soft and frustrated voice.

By the end of the conversation, both women seemed wiped out after talking about all that's happened to them. However, they both seemed to realize that because they were a part of a television story, their thoughts would soon be heard by more people than just those folks around the "coffee shop."

"I hope this helps people understand what's going on here," said Trina not really looking at me but with a stare they went right through me.

During the ride, back to the station in Toledo, there was the familiar sound of silence in the car. Both my photographer and I tried to grasp what it must be like to be so young, to be responsible for a toddler, yet not be responsible for the cancer ravaging her body. What could these kids have possibly done to deserve this? Nothing, but here we were, in the thick of ambiguity that no one ever thought would be part of their lives.

Throughout that ride, I told myself I had to get more answers and stay on top of this investigation by the state. The next day I set up a trip for Columbus to sit down for the first time with the man who is in charge of the study…Robert Indian. It was the first encounter in what would become a long, arduous relationship with Robert.

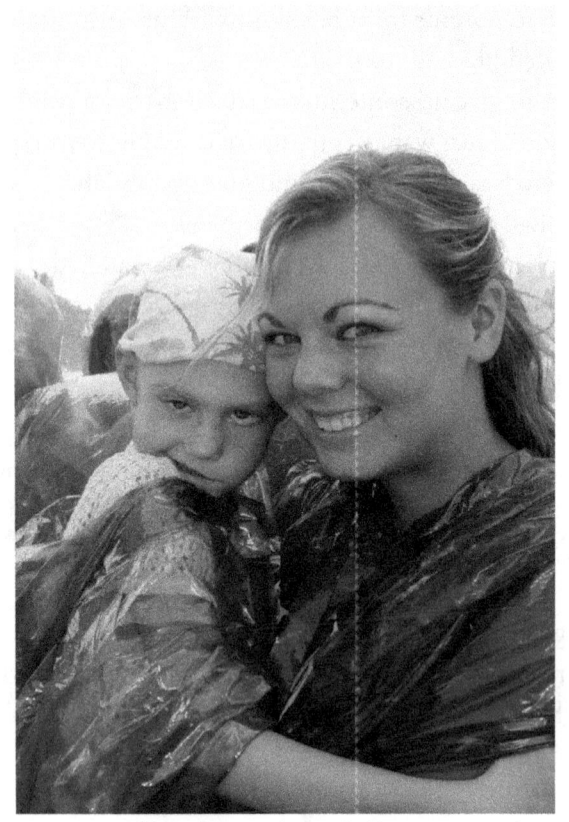

Alexa Brown, Amanda Brown

"Writing again from Buffalo New York, I read your updates every day, and am very happy you are on a break. Hope Niagara Falls is fun for you, try to ride The Maid of The Mist tour boat, as I have lived here all my life, and have never been, but am going to try before this summer is over. Just wanted you to know that my kids and I pray for you every night before bed and think about how you are feeling. Take good care! Leslie O'Leary"

Leslie O'Leary from New York
On CaringBridge.com

chapter 7

"We have to talk to this guy and find out where the investigation stands," I remember telling another photographer assigned to the case now with me. His name is Shawn Dunagan. Shawn was a shorter, slightly overweight twenty-something just barely out of college who wanted to be a sports guy. The station could only make him part-time in the sports department. When a full-time gig opened up in the news department, he decided health benefits and steadier pay would be the better way to go. Little did this Jewish kid from Cleveland know he, too, would be so compelled to tell this story.

It was a rainy, two-plus hour drive to Columbus and the Ohio State Department of Health. Water fell the entire trip down, during our stay, and eventually on the way home. Quite appropriate for the topic we were covering.

After getting to the offices of the Department of Health, a PR rep named Robert Jennings greeted us in the lobby. He was a tall, thin, black man in his 40's who had a distinguished look with glasses, clean haircut, and a sharp suit.

"Let me take you back to our discussion area," he said with a smile and waved his hand in the direction where we needed to go in the historic looking building.

He brought us to a room that looked more like a funeral home reception area. There was old carpet but nicely painted walls that had old-fashion paintings hanging from them. All meant, probably, to give a warm, calm feeling for anyone who was to have conversations about serious health matters in the state of Ohio.

The set up for the interview was right in the middle of the room with a centuries-old fireplace in the background and lots of blank space around us. Two antique looking chairs were placed facing each other. Shawn brought in the lights and put the camera on the tripod. Then, we waited.

I sat in my antique chair looking through my notes but that empty chair right across from me made my mind wander. I thought the man I was about to interview was going to be the person who would help these people figure out what was going on. I had to be on my game and ask the right questions. I have to admit I was nervous as hell.

About 15 minutes later, Robert Indian walked in. He was a short, little man with a tan leathery face and short dark hair. He wore an older-looking sport coat and slacks that may have come with the outfit.

"Our hearts and prayers go out to the families," said Robert, looking me straight in the eye. "But we also have to determine is this something unusual. Is the cancer rate higher than expected?" he asked.

At this point in the study, there were about 15 kids from a lightly populated area in eastern Sandusky County. Everyone in the affected communities there knew this was "unusual" and flat out problematic, but this guy followed the protocol for any study like this. However, as he would eventually admit years later, this case was unlike anything the state has ever seen.

At the time of our interview, Robert said he had requested medical facilities around Clyde and Green Springs to give him all reports of infants to 19-year-olds who had been diagnosed with cancer in the past 10 years. He said that information should be given to him in the next few days. It would then be up to him and his staff to determine if there was an abnormal cancerous outbreak based on the number of people living there. He told us his first review of the reported cases showed there were various types of cancer.

"That would indicate that there is not a point source or something specific playing a role," Robert told us. He went on to say that a small percentage of studies come back positive for a cluster and the chances of the cancer being caused by something in the environment like pollution or dumping were slim. "Actually, precious few have ever come back that you could possibly link to some type of environmental cause. It's almost impossible to prove," he added.

As he said those words, I thought to myself if that was the attitude going into this study, then we were not likely to ever figure this out. How in the world was the source ever going to be found?

As my thoughts swirled, I asked Robert what he would say to those families caught in the middle of this mystery. "We know we're dealing with children. We know we're dealing with parents. It's a scary time," Robert said. "We're not saying that everything is okay. We're not saying this (cancer) is acceptable. We want to see (no cases). But that being said, we know it happens," he coldly stated. "There are hundreds of cases diagnosed across the state."

That statement that gave me more insight into the thought process of this agency's approach to studies. The impression I got was that there was no hurry because they were not going to find anything anyway.

I left that interview very frustrated. I knew we were in for a long haul.

That's when I was introduced to the Brown family and a little girl named Alexa.

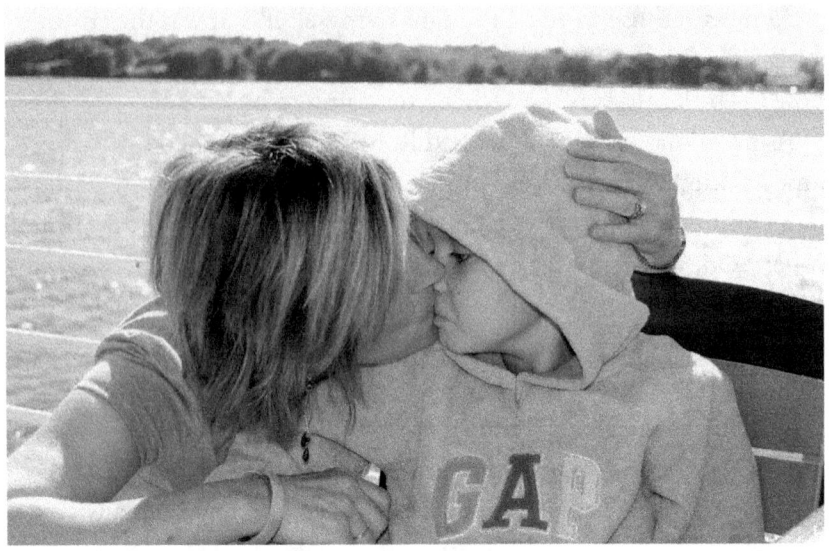

Wendy Brown, Alexa Brown

"You are not alone. Many love you and pray for you. Even here in the Hawaiian Islands, we lift you before the Lord. Aloha no Ke Akua!"

On CaringBridge.com

chapter 8

About a month went by with no word from the Department of Health, despite Robert Indian saying he would have information from the counties within days of our interview with him in Columbus.

During those four weeks, I started gathering information about Alexa Brown.

Other families told me about the little girl. Her father, Warren, was the Clerk of Courts for Sandusky County and well known in the community. My phone calls came and went without any correspondence at first. I left messages hoping to hear from the family, but understood that the holidays were right around the corner. It might not be the best time for me to push for an interview.

I finally got through. "Hello?" said the young voice on the other end. It kind of caught me off guard but I was ready.

"Hi, there. My name is Jonathan Walsh and I work for News 11."

"Yeah…" trailed the higher-pitched voice.

"I was hoping to talk to your mom or dad. Are they around?" I asked, sitting straighter now in my old, wobbly chair that could have been at the station since broadcasting was invented.

"Okay, here's my mom."

Wendy Brown was in the middle of something. To this day, I don't know what that was but I could tell she had her hands full as she hurriedly took the phone.

"Hello? Who's this?" Wendy inquired sounding distracted.

"Hi, it's Jonathan Walsh from News 11. I…" the words didn't get far off my tongue when she interrupted.

"Oh, yeah. We got your messages," said Wendy. "You'll have to talk to my husband," she added with a few more muffled words like she was talking to someone in the room. "He's right here."

Usually I had good luck making a connection with the mothers involved with this story. I am not sure why, but that was how these phone calls went in the past. When she passed the phone, I was not sure what to expect.

"Hello," said the deeper voice with a concerned tone attached.

"Mr. Brown, this is Jonathan Walsh from News 11. How are you?"

"I had a feeling you would be calling," Warren told me.

"Well, sir, I've been working on this story about so many kids having cancer and…"

"Jonathan, you have to understand this is a terrible time for our family," Warren jumped in. "I have deep concerns about coming forward with what we've been dealing with."

"I completely understand," I said, digesting the seriousness of his words.

As the conversation continued, Warren sounded like a man trying to protect his family from being exposed while at the same time wanting me to know about Alexa's struggles.

"I have to know what your intentions are, Jonathan, with this story," he told me.

"I just want people to know how awful this cancer is, how concerned we need to be, and what this mystery is doing to the community and the individual families affected," I said, hoping to reveal my goals succinctly and genuinely.

"I hope so," Warren said with a still-protective, cautious feel to his voice.

He reluctantly agreed to have me come to the house. It was December 4, 2006.

We pulled up to the Brown's home in Clyde. It was a nice house situated on a newly developed street called Lynber Lane. "For Sale" signs were implanted in the empty plots of snowy ground in front of them. The Brown home was just on the edge of a large cul du sac. It had a long front porch with a Cedar exterior and a sloped roof that hung low.

As I walked up to the door, I noticed long windows to the side where I could see plenty of people walking around. I knocked lightly on the modern front door and Warren greeted me. His appearance was a bit intimidating.

Warren stood about 6'3" with a large build. I could tell he was an athlete in his younger years. His cleanly shaved head was positioned on his broad shoulders and his frame stood tall.

As he invited us in, their foyer opened up to a high-ceiling family room with couches. To the right was a lightly colored, modern, kitchen counter that was long and about as high as my elbow. At the end of the counter, there was a dining room table where I notice people were passing by. An older child was standing to the side of one chair looking down. She appeared to be helping with homework.

The younger child in the chair was wearing a red Santa Claus hat. It was Alexa.

The Brown family is an attractive group. Abby and Amanda have model height as well as looks. Abby is the oldest child. She was the one standing by Alexa's side. Abby was in her early 20's. She had a thin build, pretty face and a smile that would make any guy pay attention. Amanda is the next oldest. She had long brown hair, big eyes, and an inherited appearance that would catch the eye of the boys. Ethan is the younger brother. He's a tall, young teen who clearly followed in his father's footsteps. He'll be playing football in no time. Wendy is the mom. She is a thin woman with shorter, dirty-blonde hair, and a talented piano player.

I am struck by yet another odd combination with this cancer cluster. Here was a family that looked strong, healthy and attractive but had to deal with such a devastating, horrible, and ugly disease. They would have traded their own health and appearance in a heartbeat to have young Alexa be completely whole again.

Alexa weighed probably 60 pounds soaking wet. She was a thin, little girl all of 8 years-old. She wore a crooked smile thanks to the tumor and subsequent surgery. The Santa Claus hat covered her bald head caused by the chemo. She was shy due to the cancer that stole the life out of her and her personality. However, it had not taken her fight.

"She doesn't complain," said Warren. "I have complained a multitude of times more than she will ever complain," the father of four added. "I am so proud of a daughter who won't just lay down and roll over," he told us with his eyes starting to show tears.

To know Alexa was to understand how she got here and why I was in her home talking to her about the battle in her brain.

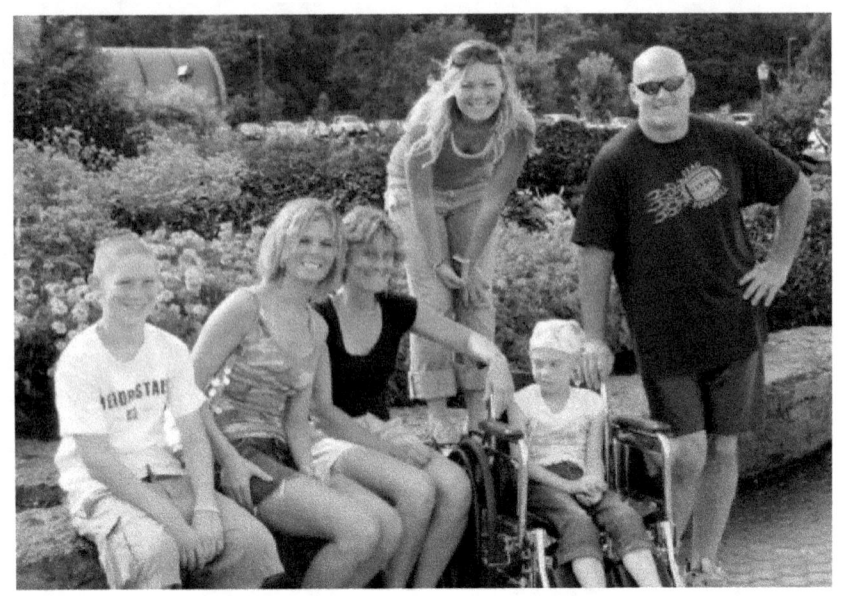

Ethan Brown, Abby Brown, Wendy Brown, Alexa Brown, Amanda Brown, Warren Brown

"Hello again...still thinking about you, pretty girl, and praying that you are feeling good today!

Wendy, I am thinking about you, too, this Mother's Day weekend. While 'have a happy Mother's Day' doesn't quite seem appropriate, I do want to say, 'thank you.' Thank you...for reminding me to look at my precious babies and see beyond the dirty hands and the whining and the messy rooms.... Thank you...for helping me to remember to read to my kids.... Thank you...for helping me to remember not to sweat the small stuff.... Thank you...for helping me to remember to cherish every moment I have with them.... Thank you...for entrusting me with your beautiful little girl. I treasure the time I spend with her, and I know I am a better person because of knowing all of you and walking a small part of this journey with you. Thank you.... for giving the rest of us mothers something to strive for! The love, strength, patience, and courage you show are truly inspirational. My wish for all children would be that they could all have the family that Alexa is so blessed to have. I do wish you happy times this weekend, and the prayers will never cease. I love you guys!"

Linda from Ohio
On CaringBridge.com

chapter 9

"Dr. Diller allowed me to cut the cord," said Warren with a slight tilt to his head and a look as if he was envisioning that precious moment. He sat back in one of the kitchen table chairs. These same kitchen chairs were the ones Alexa spent hours in trying to relearn everything the surgery snatched away from her.

"She was a normal little baby," he added. "Normal size, normal everything, and beautiful," he continued with a bit of a smile now on his cocked head and a far-off stare in his eyes.

"At home, the two older girls sure wanted to be little mothers," said Warren about older sisters Abby and Amanda. Little did they realize how much care Abby and Amanda would really have to give in Alexa's later years.

Wendy, who sat across the small kitchen table, started to remember Alexa's toddler times. "A little showoff," she said with a smile. "Not afraid to be in front of everybody," she recalled. "From the time she was a toddler, she was ready to be a leader," were the words that came out of Wendy's mouth. She sat straight up in that chair demonstrating the way a leader would sit. "Not shy at all," she emphasized.

During those toddler days, Alexa had dirty blonde hair, blue eyes, and a light complexion that would always get tan after spending hours playing outside in the summer sun.

Those active summer mornings, afternoons, and nights would find Alexa doing cartwheels and other gymnastics without ever having a lesson. "I was a gymnastics teacher for years and taught lots of kids to do back walkovers and cartwheels," said Warren. "Alexa just did them. Never needed any instruction."

Wendy told me, "Alexa was never afraid; never afraid of anything."

She explained that it was not as if Alexa would touch a burning flame, but she was never afraid of trying something new like climbing a tree or getting into some sort of adventure.

She was part tomboy and part animal-lover. Alexa would wrestle around with her brother Ethan or take on dad with a playful taunt. "I'd say, 'You wanna fight?' and she would put up her fists," remembered Warren. But her heart was also very tender. She wanted to take care of animals, not just pets but wild animals.

"At the sight of a hurt animal, she would want to fix it," Warren recalled. "I can remember her saying she wanted to be a veterinarian."

By the time her early elementary school years came around, anything and everything outdoors kept her busy. However, she also showed an interest in singing in the Junior Choir at church. Wendy was the music director. "She couldn't read, but she could memorize a song," said the proud mom.

With all her outside interests, Alexa still managed to pay attention to her schoolwork. She was always more into reading and writing than math, but she still got A's in everything. In fact, Randy Stockmaster was Alexa's first grade teacher and Wendy remembers him saying Alexa was the smartest student in class. "No offense to other families but she just was. She would read all the time. Read, and read, and read," said Wendy. "Lots of books."

By her second-grade year at Clyde Elementary, she had spent a summer full of riding her bike, doing gymnastics all over the neighborhood, and roller blading up and down the street. In her class, she was the fastest runner with an athletic build; as strong as any athlete her age could be.

All of her interests and accomplishments gave her confidence. Yet she had and an uncanny understanding, especially at a young age, of when to be or not to be in the spotlight.

"She was very dramatic, but didn't need to be the center of attention," said Warren. "She was always willing to become the center of attention. There's a difference," Warren pointed out. It would be her second-grade year when the attention she received was the kind no kid, no family ever wants.

Some weeks before the springtime, Warren and Wendy said Alexa would complain of headaches here and there. They did not keep her up at night. They were occasional and didn't last long.

Her brother who was 13 at the time, did mention a couple of times to Wendy that Alexa's eye was doing something "funny." Wendy didn't think anything of it at the time.

"She did say to me, 'Mom, I'm seeing double.' She would be sitting there doing her homework," Wendy explained. "I just thought it was because she was a studier. She would come home first thing from school and sit at that counter and start working on her homework," she continued.

There was one other time Wendy remembered that Alexa was at a birthday party and she had thrown up. She had not been sick earlier, but she had been running around a lot, eating lots of birthday treats, and baking in the hot sun. The thought of cancer certainly never crossed their minds. One day in May would change all of that.

It was a sunny and clear afternoon. Wendy had just started working in Lakeside, OH as a recreation director. Warren was at home with Alexa who was sitting in front of the TV.

"I see double," Alexa told her dad.

Alexa walked over to the chair as Warren worked in the kitchen. "She was looking right at me and her left eye wandered all the way into the bridge of her nose and came back out," he said.

Warren immediately called Wendy at her new job.

"Something's wrong with Alexa!" Wendy remembered about that conversation. "So, I came home." It was the last day she would ever be the recreation director. She never went back.

The next day they took Alexa to her longtime pediatrician Dr. Diller. The Browns thought there was something wrong with Alexa's eyes. That was it. They were a little nervous as Alexa sat on a typical doctor's office table and Warren and Wendy sat nearby in the small examination room.

"Hi, everyone," said Dr. Diller as he walked into the room. "How are things going?" he asked. The family told him Alexa was seeing double and that Warren had seen her eye wander in and back out again the previous day.

Dr. Diller did not seem alarmed, but the Browns said he would not have reacted alarmed anyway even if he had been. However, a simple test would alter the tone of the room in a hurry.

"He told her to put her heel in front of her toe and she couldn't do it," said Warren. "This was a kid who could walk on a balance beam, who could do a backbend, who could do a perfect cartwheel, but she couldn't put her heel to her toe?" Warren questioned in his head as Alexa struggled with the test.

Dr. Diller's demeanor turned serious. "We have to set up an MRI right away," he said. In fact, he ordered the technicians to do the test through their lunchtime because he needed the results immediately.

Warren knew it was not good. "I did not want to get her alarmed," he thought. As for Alexa, it was already too late. "She got really quiet. Very, very quiet," Warren noted.

After the MRI, all three went to hospital x-ray lab the waiting room. It was the same waiting room where they have waited many times before for routine ex-rays and lab work. This time it was much, much different.

"I remember when she was having the MRI done, the technicians didn't say anything," said Wendy. "But the second that Dr. Diller came into the waiting room and looked at me, I knew. That's when I knew beyond a shadow of a doubt that it was not good news."

The doctor told Warren to stay with Alexa in the waiting room while Wendy went to look at the x-rays with Dr. Diller.

As they walked into that room, Wendy's fear grew. Her heart raced. The ten-second walk seemed to take days as if time was moving at a much different pace. Wendy sat slowly, quietly dreading whatever words were going to pierce the room's air.

Dr. Diller delivered the chilling news. "Wendy, I've never felt so terrible having to tell somebody something like this before, but…(long pause) Alexa has a brain tumor." (This after Dr. Diller just months earlier diagnosed Tyler Smith with Leukemia.)

Wendy's heart sank. It was like her whole body left her. All she could do was grab Dr. Diller and hold onto him. Wendy's immediate thoughts turned to her baby girl. They had to go out into that waiting room and tell Alexa.

Warren sat with Alexa waiting for the news. Wendy continued in the other room talking to Dr. Diller. Alexa sat on Warren's lap. The girl who had been so energetic and never afraid of anything had to ask the scary question. "Dad, am I going to die?"

At that moment, Warren knew he could not show fear. "No, honey. You're not." He tried to reassure her, but they both ended up crying together even before Wendy and Dr. Diller emerged from the other room.

Dr. Diller delivered the diagnosis. "…I'm sorry." The words hit Warren's very soul but he was not surprised…very upset, but not surprised. Alexa did not really know what cancer was. It didn't sink in at that moment. Everyone was numb. All for different reasons, but all of it stemming from a single word: cancer. The next steps were a whirlwind from that moment on.

Wendy had to call her daughters. Wendy had no idea that Abby was at a McDonalds in Columbus babysitting two little kids. As Abby sat in a restaurant known for its Happy Meals, toys, and comfort food, she heard the details of the dark diagnosis. Abby had such a reaction that a nearby stranger at the restaurant had to help watch the two young ones as Abby tried to compose herself.

The Browns got into their Ford Expedition and the entire ride home did not produce a single word. Alexa who was sitting in the back of the car had the physical appearance of a healthy, athletic young girl. However, the inside of her body was in grave danger. Her small second-grade girl frame was in shock. She paid attention to the way her parents reacted. By the actions of her mom, dad and the doctor, she gathered that her life was never going to be the same. Her silence spoke of her new unrelenting fear.

After getting home, Wendy and Alexa packed up their things and got ready to take a trip to Toledo and Mercy St. Vincent Medical Center. Warren was left at home waiting to tell Ethan that his wrestling partner, his play pal, and his little sister had a brain tumor.

Warren was at the school bus stop. The traditional, yellow caravan slowly came to a stop. Warren could hear the kids inside talking and laughing. Ethan popped off the bus not knowing anything was wrong. Warren looked at his son…his only son…with disbelief that he had to tell him such an awful thing. Ethan climbed into the car and Warren revealed the devastating news.

"I can so vividly remember him just pounding the dashboard," Warren recalled now with tears gathering in his eyes. "I don't think he said a word. He's a lot like me. Just let me break something," Warren told me as his head sank into his chest.

Home was different now. The atmosphere inside the once active, bustling house suddenly took on the personality of a worried loved one. Quiet. Deep in thought. A lot of "what ifs" ran through their minds.

By the end of the day, the entire family made the trip to the hospital. Warren, Wendy, Abby, Amanda, and Ethan all sat by Alexa's side. Surgery was scheduled for the next day.

That night they all slept in Alexa's room and the room nearby. The uncomfortable sleeping arrangements were not going to prevent these family members from being exactly where they knew they had to be.

Alexa was being very "un-Alexa"…very still. She was not a little girl anymore. She had to grow up very quickly now and had to deal with a very grown-up situation.

The hospital room felt cold and disinfected. No one had a good night's sleep.

That morning, everyone went with Alexa as they rolled her through the brightly lit hallways on a steel-framed hospital bed. They gathered in the elevator and as the doors closed with that familiar thud, they realized this was unfamiliar territory. A silent ride took them to a tunnel that led to the operating room.

Alexa had not yet cried. Through all the scary, new situations she was having to face at the hospital, there were no tears. They did not start to flow from her tiny, little eyes until Warren told her everything would be OK.

Everyone huddled around the bed, holding hands, and placing them on Alexa as they prayed. They asked God to watch over her. They begged Him to be with the doctors as they were about to explore just what was in Alexa's brain. Time seemed to stand still: a feeling of "this can't be happening" overwhelmed the area occupied by a twin-sized bed. With a final Amen, that bed went through a set of doors…doors that would eventually return a very different Alexa.

Family and friends sat, stood, and paced in the waiting room for several very long hours. All kinds of thoughts raced through their minds while doctors operated on Alexa's head. What will she be like when she comes out? Will she even make it out? Why does she have to go through this?

After the 5-hour surgery, the family got the news about the operation. Things went well, but not smoothly.

"He told us he had to scrape, and scrape, and scrape really hard. However, he said he thought he got it all," explained Wendy.

The interesting thing was that Alexa did not look much different. She got back into her bed. She talked to Wendy. She walked on Wendy's feet to the bathroom. The family had a bit of hope even as they realized Alexa just had just survived major surgery. That hope did not last very long.

Within 24 hours after surgery, Alexa lost everything. She was unrecognizable. She could not walk. She could not talk. All she could do was cry. She had developed a form of Cerebellar mutism, a condition that zaps nearly everything away from a child who used to be able to do just about anything. It is a fairly rare condition that only affects about a quarter of patients in Alexa's situation, and she had it badly.

"No one told us that was possible," said Wendy in an angry tone. The family watched Alexa's condition turn rapidly worse.

It was not until a nurse did some research on the internet that they figured out what had happened.

"Completely frustrating," Wendy said looking back on the whole ordeal. "She couldn't see. She had no control of herself. She had no muscle function. She just kind of went limp. As soon as we could get her up into a wheelchair, she would just flop," she added.

Thankfully, she did not lose her ability to swallow. Some kids do.

Still, it was a nightmare playing out before their very eyes and one that was ruining Alexa's body.

Days turned into nights and Alexa was barely a shell of her former self. Therapists tried working with her but, in those first days, there was nothing that seemed to help the little girl. She had a scraped and altered brain. Worries of "is this what she's going to be like for the rest of her life?" started to repeat again and again in the Browns' minds.

Wendy, Amanda, and Abby slept in Alexa's room night after night. At one point, they needed a break. Wendy and Amanda refused to leave Alexa's bedside, but briefly relented to go to Abby's apartment to get a shower. That night, Warren was there by himself.

Warren had a lot of time to think as he watched over his baby girl. She was as still as he could ever remember. Days of riding a bike and roller blading down the street seemed like a very distant past, though they were normal just weeks ago.

He knew the surgery had been devastating. He had doubts she would make it through the night. He counted her respirations as her tiny belly rose and fell. There were many long pauses. At times, there were just seven respirations per minute.

"As I knelt there praying, I thought my daughter is going to die tonight," said Warren. "That feeling of kneeling by my daughter's hospital bed and watching her breaths…seven to 10 second pauses in between…then finally exhaling…then nothing again," described Warren. "There were so many times during that period of time that I thought she's not going to breathe again." God granted Warren's prayers that night. She made it to the next morning.

There was never a time when Alexa was alone. Someone was always there. Whether they sat in a chair slouched over the side of the bed getting some sleep while Alexa rested, or everyone was in the room encouraging her along the way…Alexa had company. The exhausted mother, Wendy, held Alexa's hand and dozed off only to wake up not feeling like she had ever closed her eyes. This took a toll on everyone but not as drastic a toll as the patient herself.

After nearly two weeks, Alexa started having some control of her arms and gave hand signals for things she wanted. With signs of improvement, came an abundance of recommendations from the experts to get Alexa more intense therapy.

As the recovery continued, the time came to leave St. V's in Toledo. Doctors recommended she receive care at the University of Michigan's Mott Children's Hospital in Ann Arbor.

The day of her discharge from St. V's was full of sunshine. As they put Alexa's post-surgical body into the car, they were worried. She could sit up in the car seat but they did not know if the movement of the car would send her toppling over.

She had to borrow Warren's sunglasses because the brightness bothered her eyes. It was yet another car ride filled with unknowns.

They arrived at the Michigan facility on a Monday. It was a big medical building with plenty of medical professionals, patients, and staff hustling and bustling through the halls.

Alexa's room was a double. Her roommate was a screaming baby suffering from some kind of airborne sickness. Wendy and Warren could not believe this was happening. As if the surgery had not been difficult enough, Alexa would have even more challenges to her recovery that had nothing to do with her.

Because it was Memorial Day, the doctor did not show up to see Alexa until Tuesday. By that time, Wendy and Warren had their doubts about how effective the therapy was going to be in such an environment.

Wendy described therapists that would help Alexa with a "bath." Wendy remembered they handed her a bag full of hot cloths so Alexa could bathe herself. She did not have that ability. Her body would not let her. Wendy said she felt the staff pushed and pushed with so many different therapies that within days, the Browns had to make a decision. By the end of that week, Wendy and Warren had Alexa discharged and were on their way back home to Clyde.

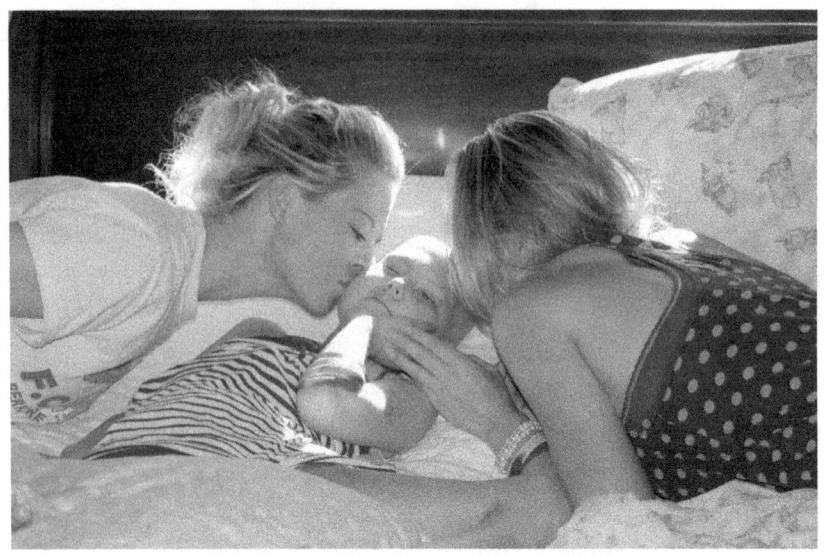

Abby Brown, Alexa Brown, Amanda Brown

"Tomorrow several federal legislators will be blitzed with faxes. 2000 letters will be faxed form student in the Clyde/Green Springs school district. On another note this family misses Alexa terribly. We know in our hearts that she is okay but we would sure like to be able to hear from her—in her voice and see her face again. We see through a glass darkly but then we shall see face to face."

Warren
On CaringBridge.com

chapter 10

Once back home, care for Alexa fell onto everyone in the family. It especially hit Wendy the hardest. For two-and-a-half years before Alexa was diagnosed with cancer, Wendy had been taking care of her mother who had become debilitated by a massive stroke. Wendy's mother moved into the Brown family home and it was around-the-clock care for the woman who had always been there for Wendy. The whole long, troubling process of being caregivers for a dying parent is anything but easy.

After a long, painful battle, Wendy's mother passed away. It was a difficult loss. On top of all that, just as things were starting to heal with Wendy, four months after her mom died, Alexa found out she had cancer. Unbelievable.

The little girl who left weeks ago to have the surgery, came home a different child altogether. Alexa's tan skin had turned a sickly pale color. The bright blue eyes that once caught attention were now distinct for a very different reason. One eye did not close correctly. The Browns said Alexa's ocular nerve was cut during surgery. And the smile that had made her dad's heart fill with joy, was now crooked all thanks to another nerve that had been severed. It still made her father feel good when she smiled, but it was just different now. Everything was different now.

It was the first part of June of 2006 and Alexa was home. She needed a lot of help to get better. "I can't even begin to describe the vocational and speech therapy that Alexa got from the members of this community," said Warren. "It was a thousand percent better than what we could have gotten at a hospital." At this point, the Browns began to include Sheryl Conley as a major player in their lives.

Sheryl has been friends with Wendy since high school. She was two years older than Alexa's mom. Now in her early 50's, she was a thin, short woman with shorter reddish hair, and thin metal-framed glasses. She spoke with a calm voice but the lines on her forehead revealed many years of worry and concern—not only for her own two boys, but also for her "adopted daughter," Alexa.

Sheryl knew Alexa since she was an infant. She watched the little girl grow up week after week at Sunday services. "I saw her at church a lot," said Sheryl. "She would be following Wendy around. She never really got far away from Wendy, but that's the way I was with my mom," she added.

Sheryl interacted with Alexa at church when Alexa sang with other children during Sunday school. Alexa participated in the children's choir with her mom. Sheryl also saw Alexa at school where she was a speech pathologist. Alexa would say "hi" and smile at Sheryl in the halls; but at that point, Alexa was never one of Sheryl's students. She did not need therapy back then.

Sheryl recalled one moment in particular that stood out in her Sunday school practice memories. Sheryl was helping guide the children in song. Alexa was 5 years old at that time.

After they practiced the songs, Sheryl told the kids, "While you're singing, if anything happens—like if I get up and run out—keep singing. Whatever you do, keep singing." The kids nodded their heads not really thinking about why Sheryl would have to step away. Alexa, however, was thinking about the reason.

A little later, Sheryl was gathering up her music and she felt the presence of someone near her. Thinking it was an adult, she turned around looking up, but then lowered her gaze found to a smaller height. It was Alexa.

"Hi, sweetie. What is it?" Sheryl asked.

"I know why you might go running out of here," the five-year-old said.

"You do?" asked Sheryl with a puzzled look.

"Yeah, because your dad just died and it's Father's Day today," Alexa said with a sympathetic tone.

Sheryl was amazed. She had not talked about that with the children. She really hadn't spoken to anyone about how difficult that day was going to be for her. She talked to Wendy later. "Did you say anything to her about my father passing away?" Sheryl asked.

"No, I hadn't even thought of it myself," replied Wendy.

This solidified Sheryl's speculation that Alexa was "just so tuned into people from such a young age."

Sheryl noticed times at school that the petite girl had a big radar when Sheryl was not feeling right.

"What's wrong?" Alexa would ask.

Sheryl thought it was funny that the tyke took an interest in her and even noticed that something was on her mind. It just so happened that things were occurring in Sheryl's life when Alexa inquired about her feelings. Alexa asked how she was on the day Sheryl's son, Tommy, was taking a big test in medical school. Then, during another day, Alexa was concerned and found out Sheryl's dog, Nestle, was not healthy.

Alexa's insightful observations happened often. "With other students, I would have just said 'I'm fine' and moved on. When I talked to any of my other students, I would talk to them as children. Not Alexa. There was something about her that just drew things out of me. She was an old soul," Sheryl described. "I never had those kinds of conversations even with my own children," Sheryl revealed. "All I can come up with is that Alexa was put on this earth for special reasons. Everything about her had to be crammed into such a short time," she thought aloud.

Sheryl recognized Alexa's intelligence and intuition. She made note of the way the five-year-old described things with her vast vocabulary. Sheryl thought, "She'll never need my help." However, one day her premonitions, unfortunately, changed.

Sheryl was in her office when Alexa's second grade teacher Sandy Cleveland ran into her room. Sandy was normally a pretty laid-back person. Sheryl was scared about what was happening that had Sandy so concerned. Alexa had not been feeling well, Sandy described. She kept Alexa out of recess.

"When the kids came back in from playing, Sandy noticed Alexa's eyes were not going in the right direction," described Sheryl. Sandy got the school nurse and the nurse called the Browns. It was right around the same time Alexa's family noticed her eyes acting differently.

Then came the day that Sheryl heard it was cancer. A sense of shock came over her body. "The first thing I thought was that it just can't be," said Sheryl. "Kids don't have cancer. My mother died of cancer, but she was older. Kids don't have cancer," she repeated. The next morning, she and her husband went to the hospital while Alexa had her surgery.

"Alexa was like a ragdoll," she remembered. It was sad to think that the once playful young girl who had inquired so many times about Sheryl's life, was now so lifeless. This whole situation was not right.

"She couldn't hold her own head up," said Sheryl. "I had just seen her at school two days before and she was running and playing. I live nearby. I could watch her run up and down the street."

As she looked at the limp little girl lying helpless on the hospital bed, the urge to run entered Sheryl's body. "All I could think was I just want to get out of there," said Sheryl quite frankly. "But somehow I held it together long enough to talk to her," she explained.

Knowing Sheryl's background in speech therapy, Wendy asked if she would work with Alexa in getting her speech back. Sheryl had all kinds of doubts.

"I really didn't want to do it. I really didn't feel qualified to do it," Sheryl said. "It's a whole different thing to be a speech therapist in a school setting than being a speech therapist in a hospital setting," she rationalized in her head.

In fact, during the time she was studying to be a speech therapist, students had to choose the clinical side or the educational side of the profession. Sheryl chose to work in schools because of one particular experience she had while doing her rotations in clinics.

"I remember working with a man who was 50 years old," Sheryl said while looking up at the ceiling and searching through her memory. "He worked for a big company in Toledo. He was one of the CEO-type people. One day he was fine and the next day he had a stroke. My supervisors were watching me through a 2-way mirror as I worked on patients. With this particular man, when he cried, I would cry," she said. "You are not supposed to do that. It wasn't that I wasn't making progress with him and getting him to do things. I would just empathize. The supervisors told me 'no more.' So, I went the academic route," she told me.

She tried to tell the Browns that she did not think she was the right fit. The thought that kept running through her mind was, "When you really love somebody, you want that person to have the best."

Wendy thought Sheryl was the best. After such a bad experience with the Michigan facility, Wendy, Warren and Alexa were ready to take the chance.

"Alexa did not want to work with anyone else," explained Wendy.

"I wanted to say no, but I couldn't say no," Sheryl revealed.

Sheryl went to work right away getting advice from experts she knew on the clinical side of therapy. She made calls and took many notes. She listened closely to what they said, then combined her experience with her students of the past. She had a feeling the Browns would not want to go back to a medical facility for all of the different treatments for Alexa. Who could blame them?

"Society as a whole has become far too dependent on the medical community to take care of their sick," Warren said citing the old adage "it takes a village." Wendy's mom had seen the same kind of focused care. "Wendy's mother would have died in a nursing home long before she did," Warren commented. "Alexa was part of that care we gave to Wendy's mother."

During Wendy's mother's stay at the Browns' home, Alexa did lots of things like play cards at the foot of her grandmother's bed and keep her company. In an interesting turn of events, Alexa spent hours playing in her grandmother's wheelchair. She went around the house maneuvering that chair through many obstacles all by herself. Little did she know, she would have to use that same wheelchair, in the same house, with the same obstacles for herself…minus the fun.

Alexa prepared for her chemo treatments in those first few days at home. She got her IV port inserted to receive the medicine that would hopefully take all the threats of cancer away.

Throughout that summer, there were constant challenges with the many therapies she had to endure. Progress was very slow. Alexa struggled to deal with her new reality but was determined to get back to a "normal" life as she soon as she could.

Sheryl stopped by the house to do an initial assessment for speech therapy. When Sheryl stepped into the house, she was not prepared to see Alexa in such a desperate state.

Alexa was lying on a big, one-and-a-half sized chair that extended out like an attached ottoman. Alexa's pale and tired looking body was just lying there with barely any life breathing through it. Alexa could not speak in a normal voice.

"The thought that came through my mind was, 'Get the hell out of here!' and I don't swear," Sheryl said after seeing what was left of the former busy, energy-filled sparkplug of a little girl. "I just wanted to turn around and run out because there was such a change in Alexa and it was so incredibly sad. There was no sparkle in her eyes. She was just kind of there," she admitted.

Sheryl not only stayed, but she made a serious commitment. She was at the house every single day, seven days a week. Her therapy started with the "you say the way I say" technique. Sheryl began with letters and numbers. There were a few she would understand, but the only things that that came out of Alexa's mouth were whispers.

The length of the sessions varied depending on how tired Alexa was feeling and how much reasonable progress was made. About two weeks into the hard work, Alexa made a small but significant breakthrough.

"S-ih-duh-n-ee," the frail girl whispered. Each individual sound when put together was her dog's name, Sidney. She loved that dog. Sheryl immediately recognized the name even though Alexa made just the sounds of the letters. Her speech was not even to the point of syllables yet—only sounds.

"It took her a long time to get out one word and she would get frustrated," recalled Sheryl. "I was constantly apologizing, but she wasn't frustrated with me. She was just frustrated with the situation," she added.

This was yet another time that no one blamed Alexa for her feelings. Those first sessions were very slow with letters, numbers, and then a couple of sounds together. It was a painstaking process day after day after day.

"I would go home thinking, 'Did we accomplish anything?'" Sheryl said about the battle. "But every now and then, there was something there, a small breakthrough, and I would put a red star in my notes. Two sounds together—whoo, hoo!"

Those two sounds became much more as Sheryl applied the additional advice from her speech therapist friends and did more work on her own. The endless hours of therapy started paying off as Alexa's voice improved. It took weeks to get a word from syllables. Even when the words started stringing together, Alexa was only able to spit out a single tone. "My little singer could only do monotone sentences, but we were getting somewhere," Sheryl remembered.

As baby steps were made, the pair tried simple songs. The "ABC Song" and "Twinkle, Twinkle Little Star" were big hits in the Brown house for a while. "They were the little sing songy songs that didn't have a wide range of notes…not too high, not too low," said Sheryl.

Eventually Alexa's monotone was replaced with a few intonations. Sheryl would get excited and shout for joy. Alexa would just shoot her a "give-me-a-break" stare. Not because she didn't appreciate Sheryl's help, but because she knew what she had been able to do before the cancer.

It was a constant roller coaster therapy ride. "On the days we made progress, I went home happy," said Sheryl. "The other days I just cried a lot…feeling like I was inadequate…feeling like these people are my friends and I'm going to let them down. There was added pressure with that," explained Sheryl.

As time progressed, Alexa read simple books, still pretty much in a monotone style. Sheryl and Alexa liked Whinnie The Pooh stories so Sheryl read the left side of the book and Alexa trudged through the right. It was reading, though, and that was important.

One day after making some decent progress, Sheryl told Alexa she was doing "Awesome!"

Then, all of a sudden, Alexa just looked at Sheryl. Their eyes met.

"I want to sing a song for you," Alexa told her teacher.

"Okay," said Sheryl who thought she was about to be serenaded by a rendition of "Twinkle, Twinkle Little Star." Alexa had put in some extra time honing that song, but she had other plans.

"She was driving last Friday on her way to Cincinnati," Alexa started. "On a snow-white Christmas Eve," she continued singing.

Sheryl knew that song. She knew it well. She waited for the chorus.

"Jesus, take the wheel. Take it from my hands. Cause I can't do this on my own," sang Alexa from her weak and frail voice. It was a far cry from the original singer Carrie Underwood whose powerful vocals have filled hundreds of stadiums packed with thousands of ears, but that didn't matter. Alexa's version filled two hearts Sheryl's and Wendy's. You see, Wendy was in the kitchen listening to Alexa. Wendy, so filled with emotion at that moment, quickly moved into another room. She feared her quiet sobbing would have interrupted the beautiful moment.

As Alexa sang, she looked straight into her therapist's eyes. Alexa had no control over her blank expression. Sheryl tried to control her reaction.

"I knew that was her favorite song," said Sheryl. "I didn't want to cry. I started physically pinching my leg so I would be distracted by the pain. It was the only way I could sit there and look at this little girl who was not blinking, who wasn't doing anything but wanting a reaction from me and I knew I couldn't cry," she described. "When she was finished, I patted her on the head and I said, 'That was awesome.' I told her I had to leave for another appointment or something. I'm not sure I even got to the front door before I started crying," continued Sheryl. "By the time I hit the car, I was sobbing. I drove home and I called my brother who has a huge faith. He talked to me for an hour-and-a-half before I could barely breathe and I kept saying to him, 'I can't go back there. I can't go back.' Then he said, 'You have to go back there.' I told him, 'I'm not strong enough. I can't do it." She did go back. She returned the next day. She had a bruise the size of a half-dollar on her pinched leg.

Sheryl brought her multi-colored flash cards with hand-written words and phrases. Some had swooping arrows pointing up to indicate inflection at the end of the word for questions like who and what. Other cards had words like "no way!" that showed a different kind of emphasis for Alexa to remember. Then there were the cards with hand-drawn facial expressions that the little girl had to identify. She certainly picked up the anger card quickly, but as she overcame obstacles on a more consistent basis, she loved pointing out the smiley face.

Alexa never got her original voice back after the surgery. Her new voice was higher pitched with a quieter tone. Definitely not as strong, but her resolve was. Eventually she remembered those inflections on the cards and started asking questions with the ups and downs at the end. It took months, but it happened. It happened during the watch of a selfless friend who doubted her own therapeutic abilities.

"It wasn't me. Being the instrument that God used to bring her back was awesome," said Sheryl.

She never did stop working with Alexa. That therapist-patient relationship turned into something so much more. It eventually became more like a grandmother-granddaughter team.

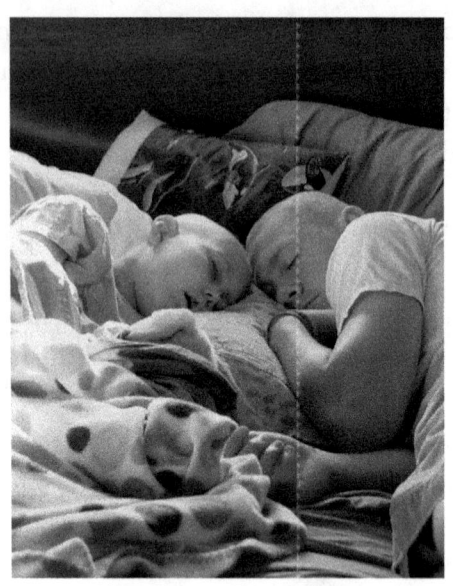

Alexa Brown, Ethan Brown

"Alexa,

I started crying when I read mom's last posting. I am sorry I cannot come and stay the entire time, but you know your brother needs me also.

Please do not allow yourself to get down too much. I saw it in your eyes yesterday and I don't know how to fix it for you. You know your dad can fix almost anything, but I can't fix you and that breaks my heart.

Lean on your mom who has been a pillar of strength for a long time. Make sure you pray for God to help you through these tough times. Go ahead and cry and scream and get it out of your system but you're only allowed to do that for a few minutes. We don't want the psychologist to think you're crazy.

Ethan and I will be down there on Sunday and I think he is planning on teasing you and making you mad so you can yell and take all your frustration out on him."

Warren
On CaringBridge.com

chapter 11

Alexa was never babied during her treatments. She was pushed with sensible expectations. In addition to the medical treatments, she had speech therapy, occupational therapy, and physical therapy that entire summer.

The therapies had started right away in June. Some of the most taxing days were those that included the chemo treatments. Her frail body already beaten-up, tried to put up a fight with the volatile drugs streaming through her blood. As tiring as the treatments were, they were an all-the-more-necessary part of the equation.

As August rolled around, it was time to think about school again. Abby moved back to Clyde from Florida after she had already gotten a teaching job there the previous year. Abby knew she had to come home to help Alexa with her education.

Warren and Wendy lobbied long and hard with the school district asking for help. After much persuasion, the district hired Abby to be Alexa's daily aide. Her oldest sister was there at school and at home helping her every step of the way.

The chemo treatments took their toll and Alexa missed many days. Having Abby by her side was crucial especially since Amanda was busy attending Kent State University. Amanda originally majored in broadcasting, but after Alexa's diagnosis, she changed her mind. She wanted to be a nurse.

When Alexa did miss school, her breakfast nook at home served as her classroom, and the table served as her desk. In addition to Abby, everyone stepped in at one point or another. Hours upon hours were spent on homework and just on life itself.

The once quick-thinking, smart little girl who excelled at all subjects now could not tackle some of those same areas. The reading that had come so easily before the cancer where the pages flew by and the math that had taken just a little more effort then, now all of it took much more time to understand. Every bit was hard.

Alexa sat at her "desk" and cried. Her short-term memory suffered. Things she had just learned with her big sis, could not be remembered a day later or even minutes later. If it was not her brain giving her a tough time, it was other parts of her body putting up a stink. When she tried to write, her hand did not flow across the pages as before. Her pencil felt like a huge tree branch and her hand like frail leaf.

Sheryl Conley was very much a part of Alexa's transition to school as well. She continued to work with Alexa on memory issues. The exercises to sharpen her recall skills were constant. It was strength building for Alexa's brain. Simultaneously, Alexa and Sheryl's relationship were getting stronger. This time it was more outside the realm of words, speech, and memory exercises.

One Tuesday while at school, Alexa felt better and bopped over to Sheryl's room. She walked up to her therapist not as a patient, but now as a friend. "What are you doing tonight?"

Sheryl was a bit surprised. While she knew the two had become close, Alexa was not one to ask for a "play-date" and certainly not with an adult outside of the Brown family.

"She never really did go over to people's houses," Wendy recalled. "When she was diagnosed, kids stopped coming over to play," Alexa's mom told me with pursed lips. It was another side effect of cancer. The disease chased friends away.

"Well, my husband is working so I was just going to go home and feed the dogs, get some supper, and watch some TV," Sheryl answered the little girl not knowing where this all was going.

Pause.

"Can I come over?" Alexa asked looking up at Sheryl.

"Well, as long as it's okay with your mom, sure," Sheryl told Alexa.

Of course, Wendy was fine with it. Soon, it started to become a Tuesday night tradition. Warren and Wendy had choral practice on those evenings and, since Amanda was at college, that meant Alexa would have had to stay home with Ethan. "I was the lesser of two evils," Sheryl laughed.

Ethan and Alexa were typical brother and sister with little fights here and there. Sheryl even used that to help Alexa in her speech therapy. "I had to work on her yelling and the best way to yell was to yell at Ethan," Sheryl told us later. "Ethan!" screamed Sheryl imitating Alexa's new found roar. "It was good for her," she joked.

"She decided she would rather spend the evenings with me," remembered Sheryl. "I guess she had a good time because she kept coming back," she laughed again.

The two definitely enjoyed their time together. They ate supper together and did homework together. Sheryl helped Alexa through some of her subjects including the speech exercises they still needed to tackle.

The new "friends" hung out, played games and painted Alexa's nails. Although, Sheryl knew that had to be done infrequently. "I didn't want to paint her nails that much because that was Amanda's area. They really liked that time together as sisters," said the mindful mentor.

They watched TV shows Dancing with the Stars and American Idol while sitting side-by-side. American Idol had a big influence on Alexa as she watched her now favorite singer Carrie Underwood win the competition one year.

The two enjoyed the cookies and brownies they made together during all of those Tuesday girl-nights. However, one evening stood out in Sheryl's mind. "Alexa was sitting at the kitchen table and I had baked a pan of brownies that we wanted to put M&M's on," said Sheryl. "Remember, we always put the M's facing up," Sheryl told the little girl who still had motor skill issues.

Sheryl thought that maybe she should not have asked Alexa to do that. "I looked over and there she is picking away at those M&M's. A lot of therapies go together. I knew she had to use her hands to grab little things just like the games we played moving people around (a game board). But I looked over and there she was struggling. I thought to myself, 'What have I done?' I was thinking, how can I get out of this so I just said I'll be over to help you in a minute," Sheryl recalled.

Alexa's response? "I'm doing fine," the little girl said never looking up. She stayed focused the entire time. She figured out how to pick up the little candies and place them on the delicious treats. Sheryl remembered this was the girl who could buzz around the neighborhood riding, jumping, throwing a ball all without a thought. On that night, there was heavy concentration needed to pick up an M&M. To this day, Sheryl regrets that particular request she made to Alexa.

There were many fantastic times the two shared baking, playing and shopping. In fact, Sheryl found herself thinking of Alexa often when she was out at a store with her husband. "I would be shopping and pick things out for Alexa like 'Oh, wouldn't this shirt look good on her or what about this skirt?' I would say to my husband Tom. He never said no." Tom knew how much Alexa meant to his wife.

"I have two boys and Alexa kind of became that little girl that I never had," said Sheryl. "Wendy was her mom. She loved Wendy so, I was more the grandmother who never had to discipline…just let her do anything she wanted," laughed Sheryl.

By this time in Alexa's life, she had no grandparents. The one grandparent that Alexa had spent time with, she watched die from the effects of a massive stroke. Sheryl was a fine "grandma" substitute. She was a person who came to be a trusted source for answers to some of Alexa's deepest questions.

As Sheryl continued to help, Alexa's entire third grade year was still more than a struggle with her mind. Her body was ravaged by larger doses of chemo. There were times her little body had to endure two-day hospital stays; then another two-day stay; then a three-day stay. Alexa could not be around anyone during that time. Her blood counts were all out of whack, her immune system was diminished, and her body was extremely vulnerable.

The radiation started taking her hair one clump at a time. "I remember a time, soon after radiation began," said Warren. "She woke up and there was a massive chunk of hair on her pillow. She just screamed."

The rest seemed to pour out. Wendy suggested shaving it off. That was one of the things that scared the little girl who had not been afraid of anything before cancer. She was afraid of losing that dirty-blonde, flowing hair that had been so much a part of her little girl appearance.

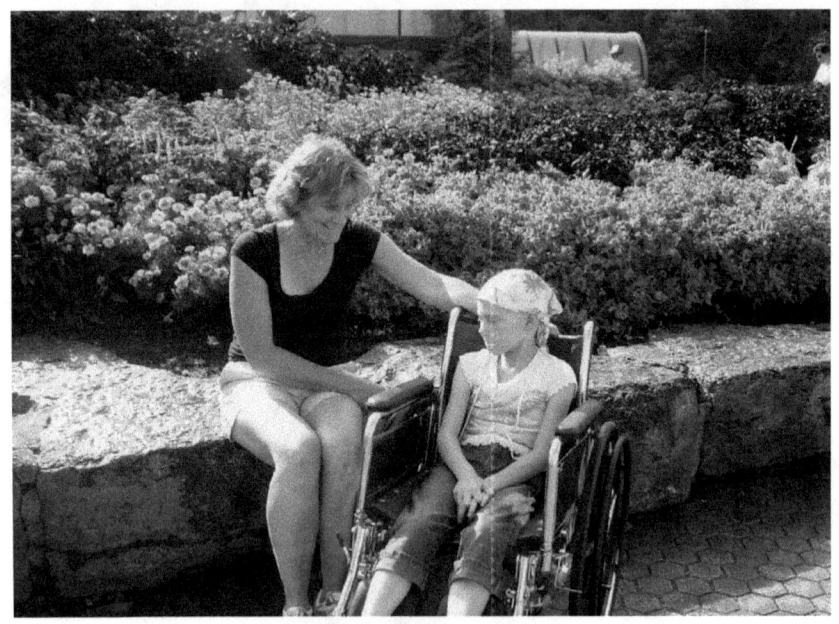

Wendy Brown, Alexa Brown

"I have often prayed that I would gladly take your place if only the Lord would allow me. Just know you are loved. I have also had cancer twice in the last 4 yrs. and Jesus has faithfully been with us each step of the way!

Again, we love you!!"

Darlene from New Jersey
On CaringBridge

chapter 12

The Santa Claus hat was a little too big for Alexa's head. She did not care. It wasn't necessarily meant for holiday cheer as much as a cover for her bald, young head.

The Christmas of 2006 was not going to be as holidays once were. There were the usual songs, decorations, and gifts like past Christmas celebrations, but the illness-ridden ghost of Christmas present was very much in the air at their home.

"I was eight years old and I found out the worst news of my life," Alexa read. Those words were from a story she wrote for a school project. When third grade girls should be talking about dolls, dancing, and pop music. Alexa's narrative was much more sobering.

"I was feeling very sad and scared," she continued. "I still am having chemo and it makes me feel tired. I just have to keep trying. I can't wait for things to be back to normal," Alexa said looking down at her paper and finishing the report.

She never looked back up. Her downward distant stare showed just how much her spirit had endured once the cancer took over her brain physically and emotionally.

"She is my role model," Abby told me during her portion of the interview. "Even though she's 14 years younger than me, she's my biggest role model." Little did I know how Alexa would become a role model for me, too. Someone I still think about nearly every day.

Shortly after our story about Alexa aired, I got phone calls from people in the Clyde community and surrounding area. "You should really check the dumping history of some of the companies in our area," callers told me. "It's got to be something in the air," others speculated. "Is whatever that caused these kids to get cancer still in this area?"

still other people questioned. That seemed to be the gravest concern for everyone in eastern Sandusky County.

It became an even bigger worry as more young children started to die from cancer. Six-year-old Kole Keller passed away in early 2007 after a long fight with Medulloblastoma, the same kind as Alexa. Kole was one of 17 kids in the study at the time. I remember writing the updated story about Kole for our newscast thinking, "What is taking the state so long?" It was THE question I heard over and over again from people all over northwest Ohio.

It would not be until May of 2007 that Robert Indian and the Ohio Department of Health finally reported this was definitely an "abnormal amount" of childhood cancer cases for such a sparsely populated region. We would also find out that Kole's family was already in contact with Erin Brockovich and her law firm about the problems happening in Ohio. There were no real details yet at that point, but we would eventually find out more about the involvement of Brockovich's firm in the years to come.

During all of this, more children were being diagnosed in and around the Clyde area. Alexa had enough to worry about in her own little cancer world, but she maintained her concern for others. There were many prayers for the community that she and the family made sure to pass along to God.

Despite the dreadful diagnosis and the ongoing fight, there continued to be at least some hope in Alexa's battle. There were MRIs taken over and over. Soon each one came up clear. The spine was good and no problems were detected in the brain. It was a crazy time, but Warren and Wendy saw a small light at the end of their lengthy, gigantic tunnel. It was a hope tested every time an MRI day came.

Warren went to work with a sick stomach the day results were supposed to come back. He tried to do his job but what-if thoughts always came back. During each instance of waiting for results, he called Wendy several times trying to get answers. When they came back clear, he gave a big sigh of relief…only to start worrying again about the next round of MRIs.

Those tests were not easy on Alexa either. Each MRI was a two-hour ordeal of lying still. Alexa had the option of conscious sedation but she did not want that. She would have to come to the hospital even earlier and stay later as was required with that kind of sedation. She wanted it over as quickly as possible so she could get back home and back to what had become her "normal" routine. For a girl who had always been active and energetic before all of this, Alexa learned to stay still amid a loud, shaking machine. The headphones full of country music helped, but so did the thoughts of going home after the test.

Additional thoughts, though, swirled around Alexa's mind. She knew she had to ask someone about them. Alexa's source for info was Sheryl Conley.

"There were times that Alexa would get a certain look on her face while we were together," said Sheryl. "I didn't know it the first time, but looking back, I did recognize when I was about to get nailed by Alexa with something I didn't want to hear." Sheryl was never taught what to say in response to some of the inquiries that came out of Alexa's mouth.

"She would always wait until we were alone together before she hit me with those tough questions. The first time Alexa got a funny look on her face and asked, "Am I going to die?"

Sheryl looked at Alexa knowing that she should not change the expression on her face. That would alarm the young girl. She tried maintaining a consistent look, but she was not sure she succeeded. "Well, we're all going to die sometime, honey, and we don't know when," responded Sheryl.

"No. I mean from this cancer," Alexa pushed on.

Sheryl admittedly was not quick on her feet. She said God entered her words that day—again. "I don't know but all I can say is I don't think so and here's why," explained Sheryl. "When my mom was sick, something told me and I kind of knew when the time was coming. And then when my dad had that pneumonia and wasn't getting better in the hospital, I kind of knew then, too. I don't have that feeling this time and that's a good thing," she concluded looking at the recovering cancer patient. Alexa bought it for the moment.

Days passed and Alexa's mind was again working overtime. That same "look" came across her face. She stared at Sheryl. "Are you afraid to die?" the tiny girl asked.

"Oh, crap!" thought Sheryl but never uttered those words out loud.

"Have you asked your mom and dad these kinds of things?" questioned Sheryl.

"Oh, I can't talk to them because they cry," Alexa said matter-of-factly.

Sheryl thought to herself, if Alexa only knew how many times she had cried when she left their many sessions together. Or the moments of tears when the worry-lined "grandmother" would be thinking about her "granddaughter."

"Well, yeah, kind of," Sheryl finally answered.

Alexa let her have it. "Sheryl, we've gone to the same church!" Alexa started saying in a bit of a lecturing tone. "Don't you listen in church? We talk about God and Heaven and what are you thinking about at church?" she rambled on while Sheryl felt the blows from Alexa's words.

"Alexa had faith way beyond what a little kid would have and beyond what most adults have," recalled Sheryl in a later interview.

During that moment with Alexa, Sheryl knew she had to explain.

"I'm not worried about what happens to me, but I don't want to leave my family," she told Alexa, referring to her husband and children she would leave behind. Sheryl also wanted to become a real grandmother, too, with grandkids from her sons' marriages.

Alexa eventually calmed down, but appeared to be making mental notes with all that Sheryl was saying.

Those kinds of talks helped. Small things like music during MRIs helped. Bigger things helped the little girl and her family deal with all of the pain and confusion of cancer. The continued support from so many people in the community kept the Browns going, too. It kept all the cancer victims' families going.

In mid-June of 2007, hundreds of people showed up at the Relay for Life event in Fremont, a town near Clyde. All around the track, people who didn't even know the families involved in the study were smiling, holding balloons, playing games, walking, and donating their time and money to the overall cause.

As I roamed the football field, among the big tents for the sponsors and the large groups of volunteers, I caught a glimpse of the smallest, but most important person of that day making her way to the track. It was Alexa.

Wearing her favorite color purple, in a little sleeveless tank top, thin shorts and a nearly baldhead, Alexa walked with a gait. She had her mom and Amanda right by her side. The faces of the two women told the story. They looked wiped out but they were happy for Alexa. Wendy had dark circles under her eyes while Amanda's eyes said, "Another year and here we are again."

After gathering a couple more shots, I made my way to a golf cart that was sitting underneath a big tree providing shade. Wendy and Alexa were sitting and Amanda was standing beside them watching the people go by.

"Hi guys," I said with a pep in my voice after noticing their tired appearance. "Great to see you again," I told them.

Alexa looked up, flashed me her crooked smile, and looked right back down. During this whole process of covering her story, I never really got the sense that she liked the television coverage, but as her parents had said, Alexa did not need to be the center of attention. She would be if she had to be. It was an important time for her to step up and keep the focus of the community on the problem at hand. This year Alexa was the Princess of the Relay for Life.

"I'm happy," Alexa told me during our interview. She looked to the side of us and noticed more and more people started to pour into the park. "They're helping everybody with cancer," she pointed out.

Another big reason she was happy that year, her body was in much better shape for the event than the previous year.

"Alexa came here like a week after getting out of the hospital last year and she was sitting in her wheelchair," said Wendy recalling the painful memory. "She had to have sunglasses on because she couldn't have the light hitting her eyes," she remembered.

This time around, while we sat together, a volunteer came by and put a tiara on her head. I could tell Alexa liked that.

"Do you feel like a princess today?" I asked.

"Yeah," she said looking down again but with an even bigger crooked smile.

"I feel touched that so many people care," said Amanda. "So many people care about her and it's very nice," she added. "How many kids are going through this right now? There's so many. Something like this can unify the community. It's very good. I love my sister," she said tearing up. "She's everything to me."

Even though there was an air of celebration at the event—a celebration of community—everyone had the bigger goal in focus: a cure for cancer. That had not gone unnoticed by Wendy and the rest of the Brown family. "Having something like this Relay for Life and all the money that goes to research and cures, is one step…one small step closer," Wendy told us during the interview.

It was an especially important step after the news that Kole Keller had passed away. The reality of cancer amongst the balloons and games was a glaring reminder. "We need to find it and get rid of it," Wendy said. "It hits home because Kole's type of cancer was the same type Alexa had. That just makes the whole situation even harder to deal with."

Shortly after our interview, all the groups of participants lined up for a parade before the race started. Hundreds of people with their matching team shirts and some with Relay for Life shirts stood together on the track talking, smiling, and holding their small children. As I looked at the crowd with the King and Queen cancer survivors toward the head of the pack, many parents pushed strollers in front of them. I could not help but wonder are they thinking, "Is my child next?"

Just then, a slow-moving golf cart started making its way toward us. We were shooting video from the field inside the track and looking toward a small hill on the opposite side of the track. As Alexa rode in the cart wearing her tiara and sporting that crooked smile, she glowed. I could tell she was into that whole environment and why not? She had made so much progress.

The cart moved into our camera shot and on that small hill in the background there was a word spelled out in large, colored cups. It was big enough to fill the mound. The word was "hope." That was what the walkers seemed to have as we took our camera on the track and talked to them. They were taking steps toward a cure.

"I'm so glad I'm out here doing this instead of being in the hospital," said the now healthy-looking Tyler Smith. She was the girl who I saw in the St. Vincent Mercy Medical Center ICU with the medical pumps around her legs. Now her legs were just fine. She walked confidently around the track. "I'm very thankful that everybody's doing this and I think it's very nice they're doing this for people with cancer."

I caught up with Chase Berger's grandmother Jane Hemmer. "There's still a lot of kids who are fighting. There's a lot of families going through a lot of stuff," she told us while wearing a dark pair of sunglasses…the same kind Chase had to wear after doctors removed a tumor from under his eye. "It's just really important to support the families. Everyone's trying to promote cancer awareness. A lot of times you don't think about it until it hits home and now it's really hit home in our town," Jane said.

As we wrapped up the day of shooting, I headed to the car and then heard a tiny voice. "Thanks for coming," I heard coming from behind. As I turned, it was Alexa smiling, waving, and looking like she had a great time. She deserved it.

"Great seeing you again," I said as I waved back and shared my own smile. "Be well," I told her. I turned back around and thought this was a good day. Definitely a good day.

All the therapies, treatments, and procedures were finally paying off for Alexa. She made significant progress and eventually finished her 15 months of chemo in August of 2007. It was time for an "End of Chemo" party at her house.

It was a large celebration. Alexa, her family, friends, and therapists put a lot of time and effort into making Alexa "whole" again. The party had more than one hundred people ready to celebrate with Alexa rather than work with her. They decorated with balloons, set up tables in the driveway to sit and visit, and swam in the family pool. Smiles were abundant even if one of them was still a bit crooked.

With every accomplishment came thoughts and hope of Alexa being a "normal" kid again. However, reality can be a bitch sometimes.

Alexa could make herself walk when she concentrated but she still had balance issues. She tried to ride a bike. She could not master it and she became scared of the two wheels that used to take her all over the neighborhood. She tried roller blading but never really had the control to get a fluid motion.

There were times when Alexa stood at the dining room window and looked across the street at the next-door neighbors who had a trampoline. Warren took her over there once, but it did not work out. She could not keep the balance necessary to bounce correctly and ever since that failed attempt, she just looked out that window at the kids. They played and ran around the yard. She stood there silent watching them with one bad eye and the other tearing up.

"I just watched her and I knew what was going through her head," said Warren. "She just wanted with her whole heart to be able to be outside like a normal little girl. She would say, 'I just want to be normal.'"

There were also times when she improvised her own fun. Alexa would go to her room and play music. She tried to dance. Her now uncoordinated body made it difficult but not impossible. That seemed to be one thing that she did not mind. Her "dancing" was one thing she enjoyed by herself in—what her family described as—"goofy" outfits. Goofy maybe. An escape? Definitely.

The summer was ending and fourth grade was about to begin. Abby accepted a different job and it was time for a new aide for Alexa. Linda Warner was assigned to her. It was an adjustment for Alexa who had been so used to having a family member by her side. Little did she know Linda would become a really close friend. The attention and focus Linda offered during Alexa's fourth grade year continues to be some of the most cherished moments Wendy and Warren remember. To think of those times now, evokes heart-rending memories and tears.

Unfortunately, there were different kinds of tears happening just across town. September was not a good month for Shilah Donnersbach who was the oldest of the study group at the time.

That summer while Alexa celebrated the end of her chemo treatments, Shilah tried to find an apartment for herself and her young son,

Nolan. Things were looking up for her until that horrible autumn day when she was told the cancer was back.

"They said it could be a week, it could be a year, there's nothing more we can do," Trina Donnersbach told me about the conversations they had with doctors. "They told us we can try experimental treatments, but Shilah just wanted to be as healthy as she could and feel as good as long as she could based on the little hope there was with any new technique," Trina said.

What had been a grapefruit-sized tumor in her pelvic area had shrunk to a baseball and then even further. However, the radiation proved no match for the angry cells. They fought back fiercely and the tumor grew more rapidly. So, did the agony.

"The pain increased so dramatically we couldn't keep up on the medication to control it," Trina explained with a heavy heart…the heart of a mother who could only feel helpless watching her daughter die.

The tumor did not stop in her pelvis. It invaded Shilah's spine and at that point it was only a matter of time. In November, they transferred her to the hospice center in Sandusky.

"They say that bone pain is the worst," said Trina. "Watching her was very…" Trina paused and tried to gather herself. "Really, really hard to watch her in that much pain."

The already emaciated young woman lied in her hospice bed wanting so much to just hold her son. The cancer denied her those moments, too.

"Nolan would want to run up and grab mommy and hug her and she would just cringe saying 'No, no, no'," said Trina, now with tears flowing down her face. "And so, he learned really quickly he couldn't even touch her."

The doctors had to give her so many drugs to try to keep her "comfortable." It's a common phrase heard around hospital beds when dealing with the final days of life. Unfortunately, the kind of "comfort" the drugs provided came in the form of hallucinations, slurred words, and a non-recognizable shell of Shilah's former self.

Trina did a lot of praying by her daughter's side all while knowing there was nothing she could do but hold her hand and encourage

Shilah. Trina needed her own encouragement because she still had to work full-time, take care of her grandson, and try to keep up with the bills. That's another thing cancer does not care about; the impact on caregivers' loved ones' "normal" lives.

Trina eventually took some time off in November and moved in some of her own things to the hospice room. She got settled in on a Sunday night, but the very next day Shilah took her last breath. Two-year-old Nolan saw her fight until the end.

"She really didn't know what was going on and Nolan was at the foot of the bed at the time just saying, 'Stop mommy's owee.'"

The young mother died at the age of 20.

"One of Shilah's fears was that Nolan would not know who she was," said Trina. "He knows that she's not around anymore, but I don't think he really understands that she's really gone forever," she added.

Trina had a picture album that she carried around in the diaper bag for Nolan. She pulled it out and Nolan pointed.

"That's mommy," Nolan said with a smile.

"That's right," Trina said with no smile.

Shilah's case was interesting in that no one in her immediate family had ever had cancer, but plenty of people living around her did have the disease in one form or another. It made her mother wonder every day. "It's so hard to say if anything at all has to do with it or it's just the unluck of the draw," said Trina with a wonderment in her voice.

During our visit, I mentioned to her that the EPA got involved with the case. It was something that Trina was relieved to hear but was upset by the news at the same time. "The EPA…that's their job is to protect people from the environment. I thought they would have stepped in to see if there really was something causing these cancer cases," Trina told me.

She planned go to an EPA meeting in January with the families involved in the study. It would not change what cancer had taken away from her and Nolan. Trina is now a mother again…a mother to her grandson.

"The toughest thing about this is doing the day-to-day stuff knowing she's gone and knowing there's still this mystery out there. I drive about an hour each way to work and that's a lot of time to think. As hard as it is to lose a child, though, it is a relief to know she is not suffering any more. The pain is gone, and she can use her leg again. She's healthy and running and doing all the things she's been wanting to do for the last two years," Trina reflected.

As we packed up the light and the camera, I headed toward the door of the old house that Trina called home. I turned around to say goodbye. I saw grandma and grandson still on the couch in the other room looking through the album of Shilah. "Mommy and doggie," Nolan said pointing to one of the pictures.

"Who's this?" asked Trina.

"Mommy has owees right there," said Nolan.

I didn't say a word. I closed the door behind me.

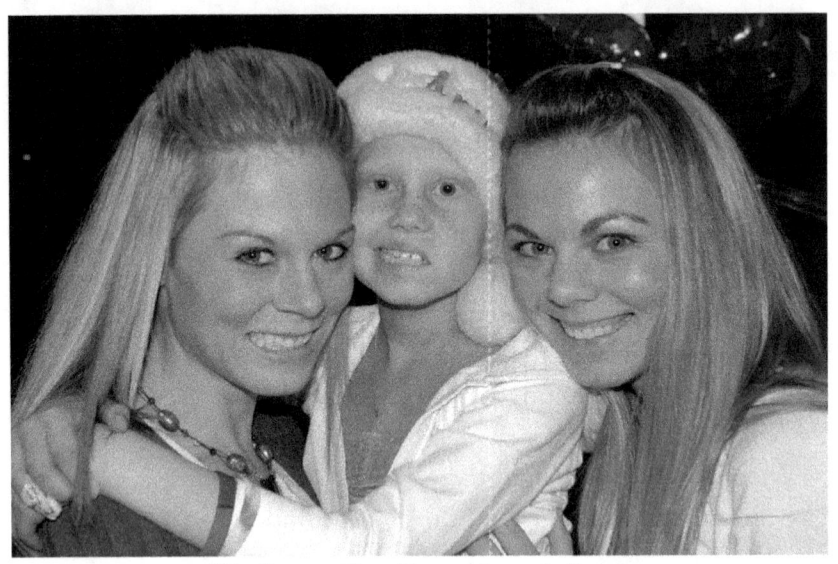

Abby Brown, Alexa Brown, Amanda Brown

"We are so glad that you had a good Christmas break and are feeling well this round. We especially know how hard this all is, but we truly believe that a good attitude goes a long way. Abby, that was such a sweet message you left Alexa. I wish, too, that we lived closer so that we could meet 'for real.'"

Denise and Alexa from California
On CaringBridge.com

chapter 13

That winter of 2008 there were closed-door meetings with the families at the Sandusky County Health Department building in Fremont. Members from the county and state health departments were there along with the Ohio EPA. Many members of the 20 families who were involved with the study at the time came to ask questions about what might be causing so many kids to have cancer. They received few answers.

The Ohio EPA provided past studies it had done concerning area companies and possible chemical dumping. However, the results kept coming back that there were no definitive indicators from their research. Plus, there were no answers from the State Department of Health. It pointed out there were so many types of cancer that it was difficult and nearly impossible to think there was a link between the cases.

I stood outside of the darkened building each time there was a meeting. I watched the family members pull into the parking lot one by one. Some said "hello" to us. They had seen the coverage during the many months and knew we tried to keep people informed.

"Here we go again," was a normal set of words I heard in those parking lots as the families walked through the front doors. Their body language spoke of the disappointment that raged through their very souls. It was a defeated looking group. Yet they were still there—still looking for answers or even clues from the people in charge of the case.

As I sat in the news truck waiting for them to come out of the private get-togethers, I was in the dark, too. Nothing from the orange glow of the parking lot lights really penetrated our car. It was cold, silent, and black. Time after time, as the family members came out from the meetings, they carried with them the same disappointment and anger.

"It's information but nothing really new," said Warren one night in that same parking lot. "I think they are trying, but it's a slow process," he added.

"What's causing this could be anything," Dave Hisey, father of Tyler Smith, said looking into our camera with his winter coat on and his visible cold breath. "It could be the cola we drink. It could be the food we eat. It could be dumping. Who knows, but we need to find out, so no other kids get this," he urged. At that point, he had no idea what was about to happen to his family in the coming months.

These meetings happened in the first few months of 2008. During those meetings, the Ohio EPA promised the families it would do more testing to help determine if something in the environment was causing the cancer cases. They were Ohio EPA promises that many in the community counted on for at least some insight into the cluster. The promises were not kept for a very long time.

Meanwhile, the Browns had almost gotten through the fourth-grade year when, in May of 2008, Alexa had yet another routine MRI. Here they went again with the MRI days. The nervousness, the worry, and the anxiety were still very much alive in all of the family members. It had eased a bit, though, since Alexa was showing so many signs of improvement.

By this time, Amanda had just finished college and was home that day. Dr. Jasty was one of Alexa's two oncologists from St. V's in Toledo. She was looking over the MRI results and eventually called and talked to Amanda. She did not have good news.

Amanda broke down but knew she had to call her parents. In tears, she told Warren and Wendy to come home right away. The Browns knew that it was usually a nurse who called with the results. So, when Amanda said she just talked to the doctor, they knew something was wrong.

Wendy had been helping a friend of hers drive to an eye appointment in Toledo but rushed to get home. Warren was at work and he, too, raced back to the house.

Wendy arrived first and Amanda barely got the words out. "Mom, Alexa's cancer is back."

It's back. This time it was in her spine.

"It was just a very sinking feeling," recalled Wendy during an interview. "She had been fine, more or less, and her tests had been clean for a while, so this was just an awful feeling."

Warren's reaction was so physical and internal. It nearly knocked him off his muscular frame. "There was always this severe anxiety surrounding the MRIs and when I heard this latest development, the feeling that came over me was I just wanted to throw up," said Warren. "I just kept asking 'What do we do now? Where do we turn?'"

After arriving home and shedding more tears amongst themselves, the Browns knew Alexa would be home soon from school. They knew they had to tell her about the cancer coming back. It was pretty much a death sentence.

"I knew once it recurs, the chances of overcoming it are horrible and that was my biggest fear," Warren told us.

Alexa came home from school and walked in the door. Immediately she knew something was wrong. The house was quiet. She could tell there had been crying going on before she stepped inside that afternoon.

"Honey, we just got a phone call from the doctor," said Wendy. Alexa's eyes started to show signs of fear. Wendy somehow managed to get the words out of her mouth even though her vocal cords were tight and her brain overwhelmed.

"Your MRI showed that the cancer is back."

Alexa sat there. She cried. She always knew this was a possibility but it certainly was not something she wanted to hear.

Wendy tried to explain what the tests had shown. "They say the cancer is in your spine. It's called 'icing' where the cancer cells are coating spots on your spine," she said, almost thinking the words cannot be real.

Alexa heard the news, tried to understand it that afternoon, but did not want to dwell on it. She moved on with dinner and thoughts of homework. It was amazing to see just how well she took it all in stride. Wendy described it as "very matter of fact" after Alexa's brief, initial breakdown into tears. Alexa seemed to have felt as if this was just going to be another fight in the battle. Everyone else knew this was a new chapter in their fight, too.

"I always thought Ethan, Amanda, and Abby had it in the back of their minds 'When are we going to get the bad news?'" said Warren recalling those days of worry and wonder among the family.

Abby had gotten a teaching job in Florida that year thinking Alexa had beaten this cancer thing and her little sister would just recover and move on. Her boyfriend's uncle lived in West Palm Beach at the time and Abby felt it had been a good opportunity to land a job and get a good start on her career. However, once the second round of cancer hit, Amanda flew down to help Abby drive back.

Here was just another example of how pediatric cancer didn't just turn patients' lives upside down. Here's a young woman finally able to start her own life away from home with a good job and a loving boyfriend whom she intended to marry. However, that all had to stop because Alexa meant way too much to miss any more moments. Cancer trumped everything, again.

The interesting thing about Alexa's physical symptoms from the cancer returning was that she had no symptoms. Her health did not deteriorate right away. She acted just the same as before and there were no outwardly significant signs that she was in trouble. The family knew, however, it was time to start figuring out the next steps for treatment.

As Wendy talked to the doctors, she was finding out there were not a lot of options. Warren kept thinking, "How can these people really not have an answer? They really don't know what to do when the cancer comes back," he told us. They searched for a good place for a stem cell transplant.

During those next months, the family had to get Alexa ready for a stem cell procedure. That meant all new rounds of chemo and all too-familiar stays at the hospital. It meant extremely painful shots. There were huge needles and lots of them went directly into her thigh. All of them tried to prepare the little girl's white cells and overall immune system for the transplant.

Besides the regular port for chemo treatments, doctors installed a Broviac line that was similar to her port, but it had two lines for the additional invasion the little girl had to endure.

Wendy's best friend since the fifth grade lived in the Columbus area. When it came time to choose Cincinnati, Ann Arbor, or Columbus for the stem cell surgery, they decided Nationwide Children's Hospital in Columbus was closer and better for the overall support of the next taxing step.

All of the grueling preparation lasted for months. The summer was filled with fear and searches for the newest, best options. Nothing good was coming up. The physical and mental toll was a price no person should have to pay, especially not knowing if all of the preparation was even going to work. It's one thing to realize the end result will pay off. It's a whole different scenario when guessing takes the place of certainty.

"That little frail girl and what she had to do," noted Warren in a later interview. "It's almost like you wish God would have taken her in an accident or something. Not that you want to lose a child ever, but she dealt with so much. Her time enduring surgeries, and chemo and radiation and all the other stuff, she never had her normal life back," Warren said stopping to clasp his weeping eyes with one hand. The memories were haunting.

The first step of stem cell transplant surgery called harvesting was unknown territory for the Browns. At the time, they had no idea that even by following the letter of the law with procedures, drugs, and treatments, the surgery could possibly not work.

"All of this opened her up to a lot of pain," Wendy said. "The machine they used to basically suck out the marrow was less intrusive than bone marrow transplants. But it was still so much for Alexa to absorb. For Alexa's type of cancer, her own stem cells were harvested. Other cancers can use donor cells."

The first attempt failed. The harvesting did not take and that meant the Browns would have to wait and try again. It was another round of bad news. Alexa did not want to add it to her already overwhelmed brain.

Eventually, Alexa got her blood counts where they needed to be for a second try at the stem cell harvesting. The procedure was successful. Soon after came the stem cell transplant.

The recovery was a bear. Because of stripping down her immune system and everything that was required for the surgery, Alexa developed sores along her throat. It was a side effect of the intense chemo treatment. She couldn't even swallow for many days because the pain was so severe.

Her throat was just one painful problem. There were several weeks when Alexa had to have special sponge-like baths because her skin was very sensitive from all that had happened. Her skin was actually a shade of brown and the medical staff had to wipe her skin in a special way with gloves the entire time. There was a fear of germs and infection.

All of this was another example of how "un-normal" Alexa's life was. She could not take a shower or a bath like all of her other friends. She could not eat with her family like all the other little girls and boys her age. She did not have the strength to play. She could not even try to get out of the room for some recreation for fear of the repercussions. Just to enter Alexa's room, people had to wear gloves. There were special transplant rooms—private rooms—with unique air filtration. It was very much not the normal life of a fifth grader, but just as she had always done, she was determined to enjoy the things normal families shared.

One of the saving graces at the hospital was Crazy Mary. She was the "Game Lady." Crazy Mary was there for the kids when it was time to do homework or to just take their minds off of what was really going on. Alexa and Crazy Mary formed a bond and became fast friends.

They started a Monopoly game one afternoon instead of hitting the homework. Monopoly sounded more fun to a child with cancer. Shocking, I know. There were times when they did have to stop and move on to the next part of medical procedures scheduled for the day. The two Monopoly moguls decided to memorize every piece of the game so when they pulled it out the next time, they could put everything as it was where they left off. It was the longest game anyone at the hospital had ever played.

To show off their commitment to dominating the world of finances and real estate, there were messages written on a chalkboard at the hospital to let everyone know how well Crazy Mary and Alexa ruled the Hasbro staple. The game was one of the only things Alexa could look forward to. It was something she did have a bit of control over and could actually have a chance at winning. Alexa loved it.

The hospital routine to and from Columbus impacted the family immensely. At one point, Amanda ended up going to the emergency room at the hospital in Columbus.

Amanda had been driving the 110 miles (one way) to and from Columbus and she was driving from home to school at the University of Toledo that was another 50 miles (one way). She wanted to be right beside Alexa as much as she could.

Wendy had been down the hall when all of a sudden, she saw a medical team racing into Alexa's room. Wendy thought there was something wrong with Alexa, but when she got to the room the med team worked on Amanda. She had heart palpitations and big problems breathing. They eventually checked her into the ER and decided her condition was related to the physical exhaustion, the worry, and stress of yet another round of cancer her baby sister had to go through. Amanda's heart is so big, but that couldn't overcome the massive repercussions or cancer hitting her family.

Thanksgiving was on the way and she desperately wanted to be home for a good turkey dinner like they had always done in the past. "She broke the record for recovery time," said Wendy. "You watch these TV programs and you have a patient get a bone marrow transplant and then 'boom' they are recovered. That is not the case at all," she continued. "But Alexa did her best that November to heal as quickly as she could so she could be home for the holiday. We were out of there with days to spare so I could make that Thanksgiving bird."

There was a lot to be thankful for during that Thanksgiving, but there was a lot still to do during the holidays. Warren and Wendy had a choice to make about radiation and whether or not to keep Alexa on the regimen that invaded her body again and again.

"I think it was a mistake when we decided we should do more

radiation because there's only so much her body could take," said Wendy. "Talking to the doctors, they agreed we should put her on the radiation schedule. I think it ruined her immune system. They thought it would be good, but it wasn't," she added with a far-off look in her eyes. I could tell she was thinking "what if" thoughts.

Warren jumped in. "Looking back, we can speculate because there is not enough research. All we can do is speculate," he told me. "It all falls back to not knowing. The reason you don't know is because no one is keeping track of it. No one is studying it enough because there's no money to be made right now."

Wendy nodded her head. "I don't think there is enough collaboration between knowing what this person in one hospital is doing and that person in another hospital is doing," she said with conviction and a bit of frustration in her voice.

Warren then told me, "At the beginning when the cancer is diagnosed, doctors have a game plan, but they're not as prepared when the cancer comes back. There's just not enough…" his statement stopped as he gritted his teeth.

Alexa ended up having 20 rounds of radiation that ended the week after Christmas. "We did what we thought was the best thing at the time," Wendy said.

"We saw some of the same people (from the hospital) that we saw the first time around," Wendy continued describing the additional treatments. "You do not think that these people will pop up in your life again. They were the nicest people, but you don't WANT to see these people at the hospital again treating your daughter who you thought was done with all of this."

In addition to the radiation, Alexa took Accutane in very large doses. Accutane was being explored to treat several types of cancer, but it was also used for severe types of acne. With that came side effects for Alexa. She experienced a drying out of her system and a peeling away of her skin. Remember, Alexa had a brain tumor and problems with her spine. Cancer ended up hitting every part of her body.

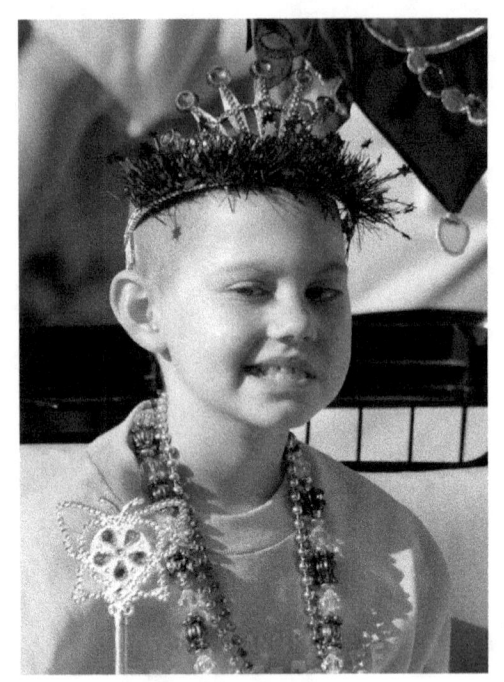

Alexa Brown

"Did anyone notice the Browns/Bengals game yesterday? They had pink ribbons and pink wristbands, etc. What about September? Where was their GOLD (the color used for pediatric cancer)? Do they have kids? Do they know any children?"

Abby
On CaringBridge.Com

chapter 14

By October of 2008, I was frustrated over and over again that nothing seemed to be getting done with the additional testing promised by the Ohio EPA. My calls to the Ohio Department of Health kept getting canned answers. "The Ohio EPA is doing the testing and based on the science that's where we will turn," was the standard statement.

I asked about the testing being done. The Department of Health reps kept telling me to ask Ohio EPA. The agencies were not working together as much as they should. In fact, after hanging up my phone one day in the newsroom, I wondered if they had ever kept in touch during the past eight months since those private meetings with the families at the Sandusky County Health Department building in Fremont.

"I'd love to be able to ask you some questions about your involvement with the cancer cluster study," I said over the phone to Dina Pierce, who was a spokesperson for the Ohio EPA. "Can I come down to Columbus for an interview?" I asked.

"Well, it just so happens I will be in your area next week for a presentation on something else," Dina told me. "You can cover that event and before the meeting we can sit down and talk," she added.

"I'd like to get you on camera for my report," I told her.

"Sure. No problem," she answered.

After our discussion on camera that day at the event, here was the report I filed for the 11 o'clock news:

"A Northwest Ohio family is going through another nightmare," said our main anchor Jerry Anderson. Jerry was a journalism veteran, the most credible anchor I had ever worked with, and could easily have been on CNN at any point in his career. His delivery was strong. His voice was perfect. He had decades of experience with northwest Ohio. It was his home and had been since he was a child.

"After one of their children has gone through a fight with cancer, now another child has been diagnosed," Jerry said into the studio camera. "It's all part of a more than two-year long medical mystery in and around the Clyde area. Jonathan Walsh has been following this story from the beginning. Jonathan, where do we stand with this cancer cluster?"

I was in the studio with scripts in hand. I was a bit nervous because I knew once this story got out, it would cause quite a bit of controversy between the community and the state agencies in charge of the study. However, I was confident everyone needed to know what was really happening, or not happening (for that matter) with the very people who were supposed to be looking out for the good of eastern Sandusky County.

"That's a great question," I answered Jerry. "The State Department of Health has already determined there are way too many childhood cancer cases around Clyde for that population size. The Ohio EPA is now involved, but the families are questioning what's really being done while more children are dying and others are added to the case list…added like the Hisey family…again," I said as the director rolled the tape of my recorded report. Here we go.

"Pretty shocking…something we weren't prepared for," said Dave Hisey in a hospital room. "We thought we were all done with all this," he added with a very concerned look on his thin face.

My recorded voice came up, "Dave Hisey and his family don't understand why after their teenage daughter Tyler Smith went through a life-threatening battle against leukemia, that now their 10-year-old son Tanner Hisey has been diagnosed with leukemia as well." The whole time I was speaking, the report showed the skinny little kid that was Tanner. He had a normal height for his age, but he was a very thin, young man. He had his shirt off while sitting on the examining room table. His short blonde-brown hair was cut tight to his head and he had the biggest eyes that even those who didn't know him could tell were full of fear.

"I look at him and think he's got his life ahead of him and it just crushes me," Dave told our camera all while getting tears in his eyes. "It crushed me for my daughter and it crushes me to think of what he's got to go through," he continued, staring off camera and right at his son just a few feet away on the table.

"How are you feeling?" asked the female doctor wearing her traditional white lab coat and a stethoscope around her neck. She began her exam.

"Tanner is in the same hands of the doctors who helped his sister at Saint Vincent Mercy Children's Hospital," I said on the tape.

"Deep breath," the doctor asked as she pushed her fingers into his abdomen. Tanner winced. "I know you don't like that part," she acknowledged.

The report then showed file video we had of when his sister Tyler was in the hospital. In the pictures, Tanner was sitting at the bottom of her hospital bed playing Candyland with Tyler and their younger sister, Sierra.

My voice continued on the tape. "Tanner was there playing with his sister a couple years ago as we watched Tyler go through her fight. What does he think of his diagnosis now? He's worried," I noted.

"If I get sick, it will be really bad during this battle and I don't want that to happen," said Tanner. "I don't like having to go through this at all."

My narration continued. "Tanner is now one of 20 children who are part of the Clyde area study. Two children who were a part of the case have died since the mystery first unfolded more than two years ago," I said as pictures of Kole Keller and Shilah Donnersbach appeared on the screen.

"After the county and state health departments could not find a common link to the cancers, they brought in the Ohio EPA," I told the viewers. "That agency met with the parents for the first-time last January and then again in March. News 11 wanted to know what the EPA has done since those initial meetings," I said.

"Without a specific direction to go, we're just trying to find anything," said Dina Pierce. Dina was a heavier-set woman with older looking glasses and brown shoulder-length hair.

The report continued with my voice. "Dina Pierce is a spokesperson for the Ohio EPA. She says the EPA's role is to support the investigation and reps have looked through records of companies, and walked through their buildings to see if anything is suspicious with emissions. But families want to know, what about actual testing?"

The next shot of the report shows Dina on the screen and you can hear my pointed and aggressive questioning in the background. "Have you tested the air? Have you tested the water? Have you tested the soil? What's been going on in the past six to seven months?"

Dina had a blank look on her face as her round glasses sat on her nose. "We haven't run any of those kinds of tests," she admitted to me.

My voice popped up again with a paraphrasing of what Dina told me in the interview. "Pierce says the EPA is trying to establish a meeting with all the agencies involved, even having a conference call last month to set that meeting up, but nothing has been established yet."

I remember as I was voicing that part of the story, I thought to myself, "I can't believe these government agencies. They have meetings about meetings. They talk so they can talk later. They have studies about a study and yet they're so busy in their schedules that they can't get together and talk about why so many children are getting cancer and why they're dying from it?" It's unbelievable, unconscionable, and just plain insulting.

Despite my disgust, I had to be fair and tell our viewers what the EPA was doing. My voice continued. "Pierce says the EPA has not forgotten about the families and the case is a high priority." However, I wasn't about to let that go. The shot on the screen is back to Dina and my insistent voice again asking in the background. "When these families hear 'high priority', they're going to wonder 'OK, if it's such a high priority, why haven't we done anything in the past…as far as testing and ruling things out…why haven't we done anything in the past six to seven months?'"

Dina looked a bit scared but, much to her credit, she did not try to make anything up. She just told the truth. "Um…I can't answer that," she told me.

I told people in my report, "Pierce explains there's a lot of work that goes into tests like that before physically doing them." All the while, I felt the agency had plenty of time to get that process going.

"It's not a fast process unfortunately," said Pierce in my story. So, I continued her "unfortunate" theme:

"Meanwhile, **unfortunately**, families like the Hiseys have wondered should they have been doing something differently all this time," I said on tape before the viewer heard this from Dave Hisey. "The two years it's taken to do this study, my son's gotten sick," he points out. "So, did I let him down? Did I let other people down by not pushing the EPA or somebody to do more?"

Before I go on here, I have to stop for a moment and ask something. Can you even imagine why a father who, through no fault of his own and who has two children with cancer, is even having to ask this question? Why in the world should he have to beat himself up over this?

Back to the story and my "unfortunate" verbiage continued. "Meanwhile, unfortunately, the city of Clyde is having to put on fundraisers for the families. Don't get me wrong. They want to help the families. They just wish they didn't have to under these circumstances," I said as the video showed a local school filled with people having a chicken dinner and auction called "Team Up for Tanner."

"It's very important," said a father named Gary Tuckerman, who sat with his loved ones in the school cafeteria eating the fundraiser food off a paper plate. "I have two kids of my own. We don't know what's going on. Hopefully, we find out what's going on in Clyde," he told our camera.

Just then, shots of Alexa Brown appeared in my report as I said, "The Brown family wants to know, too. Alexa Brown, who News 11 has featured before as part of this cancer study, UNFORTUNATELY has seen the cancer return. This time in her spine."

The pictures showed Alexa in a thin white sweater and a bandana around her bald head. She looks tired and sickly, but she was still there in that cafeteria supporting others who were in the same boat she was. She knew how important it was to show up to these events even if it was too late for her. She constantly thought of others before herself and I would later find out just how much that really was the case.

"We've run into them at the hospital several times in the past month-and-a-half," said Wendy Brown who also looked wiped out with even deeper, darker circles under her eyes and looking like she had lost weight on her thin frame. "And we just want to support them," Wendy added.

My narration took a sympathetic tone as I said, "The Browns and the Hiseys can't say enough about the people of Clyde during these tough times."

Amanda Brown then pops on the screen. "They care. They really do," she said sitting at the very tables where hundreds of other people knew her sister's story, too. "They cared when Alexa had her benefit in the summer. My friend, Emily, just had a benefit for Alexa and there was a big turnout. We are just thankful," Amanda added.

"Thankful, but also mindful of what this mystery is doing to the community and the children who are not cancer patients," I recorded on tape.

"I just wish all of this would go away so everyone can have some fun," said Tanner sitting on that cold, doctor's examining table.

He ended the taped version of the report and then it was my turn to wrap up the story back in the studio.

"The Sandusky County Health Department says it remains the lead investigative agency on the case. It's brought onboard a group from the CDC that specializes in toxic issues to help. The Ohio EPA says the Clyde cancer study is the only one of its kind that the agency is working on. The families are looking for action. I'm Jonathan Walsh… News 11."

My report sparked outrage in northwest Ohio. People from communities all over the area wanted to know why testing was not being done. They called our newsroom. They emailed me. They sent me letters that vented their frustration, but no one took it as far as Margaret Douglas-Garcia and her mother.

Margaret saw my story and the next day she and her mom, Christine Bell, set out to get a petition started. "I feel really bad this is happening to these people and it could happen to me and my family tomorrow," Margaret told me.

The petition was to force the local government to push harder for answers and actions. Margaret did not know the families involved but she has loved ones in and around her community of Sandusky County. She wanted to protect them and their future.

Margaret and her mom were aggressive about gathering the signatures. Her mom stood in front of the Clyde public library asking for support from the people walking in. She said that at one point, security and the librarian forced her off the property. By the way, it was public property, so she stood on the sidewalk of the library. The sidewalk was about ten yards from the entrance and parking lot. The "authority" figures then threatened to call the police on her.

"So, I told them, a year from now if we have 30 cases, you guys remember I was here trying to do something about it," said Christine.

It was hard to believe people would not understand the goal of helping children and helping a whole community, but that was how the women were treated.

A few days later, I found myself standing in front of Clyde's City Hall in the heart of town. Our news van was set up. The truck had the tallest mast in our fleet. I waited for Margaret to show up to do a live interview for the 6pm news. She had gathered hundreds of signatures and anonymous tips about possible causes of the cancer in the community. She was about to present all of it to the Clyde City Council that night.

Margaret was a shorter, dark haired woman whose appearance was usually reserved. However, she was not reserved when talking about this issue. "I just want them to do something about this and get the testing done," she told us. "I couldn't believe it when you reported that no extra testing had been done yet. That's why I started this petition. They need to see this," she added. "We've got to do something to make it what it was—a pretty little town," Margaret said during our interview.

I told people that night if they had any concerns that they, too, should come to the meeting and boy, did they ever.

After getting a bite to eat at the local "Italian" restaurant that was more like a sub shop with lasagna on the menu, I headed into council chambers. It was a packed house with standing room only.

The tiny room had rows of seats filled with people I recognized including the family of Chase Berger and even Chase himself. Dave Pollick, who was the Sandusky County Health Department Commissioner, was sitting toward the front. Other city employees were scattered in the crowd of agitated-looking people.

The council members called the meeting to order and got right to the concerns served by my report. The half-circle of people in charge had a mixture of men and women who all looked professional, but they still had a hometown feel to them.

Margaret was the first to be called. "I was so concerned after the report on News 11, that me and my mother went out and gathered these signatures from people who were also concerned and frustrated with what's not being done," she said holding up the stack of papers in her left hand. "Then I got these anonymous tips from people in the community who have lived here a long time. Some have guesses about what might be giving these kids cancer," she explained. "We ALL want you to make sure the state and federal agencies are doing their jobs," she told the council in a firm but respectful voice.

One by one, other community members approached the microphone. They all weaved in and out of the huge crowd to position themselves up front. They voiced their disappointment in the lack of progress and in the council for not being on top of what had become the single biggest challenge the community had ever faced.

As the meeting rolled on, more and more people showed up filling the room with additional concerns. Voices were raised several times, including a man wearing overalls from the city's water department who took issue with our report.

"I saw what was said on the news and I have to tell you it's not the truth," he shouted from his seat that was directly in front of where I was standing. "I work at the water plant and I can tell you we have to do testing on that water and report those tests to the EPA. So, if they're saying testing isn't being done, that's just not right," he screamed.

I couldn't help myself. This guy had taken my report personally and never heard the full gist of what the Ohio EPA admitted. The agency was not doing additional testing on anything when it came to water in wells, ground water, or water in the rivers or streams.

"The Ohio EPA admitted on camera it's not doing the testing, sir," I pointed out to him. He never turned around. He only put up his hand to me and waved me off like I was crazy. Yup. I was the one who was crazy.

"I find it disturbing, Dave, that there hasn't been testing," said Councilwoman Carolyn Farrar addressing Dave Pollick. "Why are we waiting?" she inquired.

"We're getting a little more action from the Ohio Department of Health and the Ohio EPA," said Dave alluding to a mid-December meeting that was newly scheduled in Clyde. Local and state agencies would meet as a result of our latest expose' on the lack of action.

It was the meeting the community had been waiting for. It was a shame all the citizens had to wait so long.

It was in the middle of December of 2008—at the same time when Alexa had already gone through the stem cell transplant and was into her 20 rounds of radiation following that surgery. The Clyde High School auditorium was filled with anticipation, anger, and tension. People from all over northwest Ohio came in their winter coats, hats, boots and gloves to sit and hear what the agencies had to say for themselves.

The row of about 10 "experts" and government reps lined the stage opposite the rows of people staring straight at them.

It was amazing to hear the same words over and over again from the people in charge of the study about how "committed" they were to this study. They supposedly had done so much work already looking at data from various companies and dumpsites. It amounted to a rehash of things these people had already heard.

One by one, the reps talked about the science involved and how long it takes to investigate. The broken record was just about to be repeated again when, suddenly, the director of the Ohio EPA, Chris Korleski, said the childhood cancer cluster was going to get top billing. "We are making this our number one priority in the state," he said, trying to reassure the community members the state was taking this seriously. He also said that, within the next 30 days, agencies would begin monitoring air and drinking water samples to try and find possible cancer-causing chemicals.

After so many broken promises, however, the people were very, very skeptical. "It's time to either rule some things out or find what's going on and give people some peace of mind," said Dave Hisey after the meeting.

By the end of the month, the Ohio EPA established a website that promised to keep people informed about the testing. It would give citizens updated information about the cluster research.

Later that winter, the Ohio EPA announced it was doing sample air testing in Clyde. We were there with our cameras as the devices were placed on rooftops. They would remain there for an entire year. Yes, it would take yet another year of gathering tests before they could be analyzed and any results given. Another year. Alexa Brown did not have the luxury of another year.

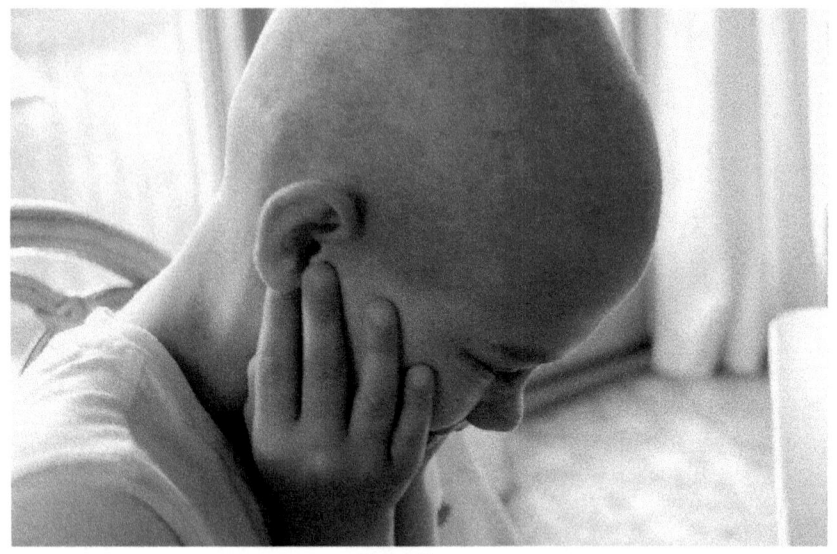

Alexa Brown

"I spoke with your mom a couple of days ago and she told me how well you're doing. Don't worry about your hair. When I was little my father had my head shaved because I had so little hair, he thought it would grow back thicker! My mother wasn't too happy he did that, but everything grew back fine!

Lots of love,

Ronnie Drakert from New Jersey"
On CaringBridge.com

chapter 15

Following her stem cell transplant, Alexa had been attending school through January, February, and March. There were challenges, but Alexa fought through them determined to be like every other kid going to class. The problem was, not every other child had the war wounds from cancer or the continued deterioration they were accomplishing.

Easter Sunday of 2009 was in the second week of April that year. The Brown family headed to church and Alexa wore a nice blue dress and a white sweater. During the service the Browns sang and prayed for new hope in Alexa's fight. The church pews were filled with the weekly faithful and those who just went on Easter and Christmas. All seemed to be on the same page, though. As people sung the hymns, you could see eyeballs stealing glances at Alexa, knowing how the little girl had struggled.

The day was perfect with Easter baskets, colored eggs and a nice family meal. They enjoyed the holiday known for Jesus rising up, but on this day, it was another step toward Alexa's downfall.

That night Amanda told Wendy, "Alexa says her legs hurt." Wendy did not know what to think of that, but she did know it was something they had to look into.

They made an appointment at the hospital. Another appointment. There was supposed to be an MRI in the middle of May, but they moved it up earlier after doctors heard about the sudden pains in Alexa's emaciated legs. It was another hurry-up-and-wait scenario. They rushed to the hospital not knowing what was wrong then waited for the test results.

Eventually the MRI showed Alexa's worn out spine had succumbed further to the cancer cells. It was spreading. The cells multiplied. The pain increased.

There were times when Alexa was fine if she was helped to the sink to brush her teeth. She could stand there, but after a little while, even that was not possible.

It got so bad it was time for a wheelchair. Alexa hated it even though she used to play with one when her grandmother was sick in their home. This time the cold, metal seat was for her.

She had to go to school and wheel around the halls; the same hallways where she used to skip around, chase friends, and walk from room to room. There were times when Wendy had to carry Alexa into the building. It was painful both physically and mentally for the little girl.

"I remember there was a day when her class was going to the Rutherford B. Hayes Museum Presidential Center in Fremont," said Wendy. "Amanda drove her and spent the day with Alexa. There's a picture of all the kids on the steps and there's Alexa sitting in her wheelchair," she added with a distant stare again remembering the picture as if it were right in her hands—so vivid, so telling, and so heartbreaking.

It was early May of 2009, and Alexa was not doing much better despite the treatments and tremendous efforts of the family and local doctors. The traditional techniques of attacking the cancer that had spread through her nervous system were just not proving effective.

The family asked all kinds of questions about what drugs were available. Doctors gave them options. They were expensive options.

Warren often battled the insurance company about what would be covered. He knew the discussions would not go well, especially when the drugs were $25,000 each. The insurer told him some of the drugs would not be included in their plan and the family would have to find a way to pay.

"I told them, 'OK. Don't cover it. You'll see my face plastered all over Toledo news!'" It's important to note, Warren is not a man who throws his weight around and takes financial advantage of the attention he and his family were getting because of this public fight. However, his little girl was not walking, not getting better, and was dying right in front of his eyes. What choice did he have? The insurance company eventually agreed to cover the treatment after it found a different drug that was an adult drug for the young girl to try. The Browns heard it MIGHT work.

Meanwhile, the family scoured the Internet trying to find something that would help the 11-year-old girl. There was a drug trial here, an advanced study there, and maybe an in-hospital stay somewhere else. Each had certain criteria that had to be met with exact specifications for each patient. The endless hours on the computer with the screen's glow radiating off their faces gave them no solid options.

About the same time, Alexa's speech therapist and "grandmother" was chosen to help Alexa prepare for the state's standardized testing in school. Alexa did not want to take it and, quite frankly, Sheryl did not want to give it to her. However, rules were rules no matter how much they didn't make sense, thought Sheryl.

Last year during the same time of the school year, Alexa had been doing well and the tests were not that big of a deal. This year, her fifth-grade year, that was not the case. Sheryl had to become Alexa's "scribe". Sheryl could not read for her but could only write the answers Alexa gave. Overall, Alexa was not feeling well and Sheryl knew something was progressing with the cancer.

On the second day of testing, Alexa had a strange, grey color to her face. It was similar to a person who was not getting enough oxygen. Sheryl recognized that look. Her mother had that same color towards the end of her battle with cancer. Sheryl was scared.

"Are you okay? You breathing okay?" asked Sheryl with a tone that did not fully reveal how terrified she was. Alexa did not really respond. She just wanted to get on with the testing.

The previous day Alexa was reading the questions out loud. "You're really going to get bored just sitting there if I don't read these things out loud," said Alexa to Sheryl. Again, she demonstrated how she would think of others. However, on the second day of testing, there was a dramatic downturn.

Alexa's greyish face just stared at the booklet. She picked it up, looked at it some more, and did not say a thing. Nothing. She looked at it, then looked at Sheryl, and then looked back to the booklet. Her grey face was expressionless. Sheryl thought Alexa was seeing double or something else was just terribly wrong.

"I first looked around the room to see if it was bugged," Sheryl told us later. "I just decided to help her a little bit," she recalled.

Sheryl decided to read a question and told Alexa to give her an answer. Nothing. The questions were easier in the beginning of the booklet and then got gradually harder as the tests went on. These were the easier questions, but they did not seem easy at all to Alexa.

None of it made sense to Sheryl, yet she could not show her concern. "Well, we can just skip the ones you don't know and we can come back to them later," she told Alexa with a positive tone. "I kept reading, one after another and Alexa kept answering, 'I don't know. I don't know.' She couldn't think and she couldn't read. I didn't know what to do. Then we were skipping pages, not just individual questions," she added.

Then, as if a switch was turned on, Sheryl noticed the color had returned to Alexa's face. It was 45 minutes into the testing. "She picked up the book and started reading and giving me answers," Sheryl recalled in amazement. "Here we were several pages into the test. The questions were getting more difficult and all of a sudden she gave me an answer," she continued.

Sheryl then told Alexa they had to go back to the previous questions that Alexa had skipped. "I did?" the little girl asked. Alexa had no idea. She drew a blank about the previous 45 minutes. She was not aware of what had just happened.

That afternoon while Alexa was in the restroom, Wendy arrived to pick her up. Sheryl had to share the 45-minute lapse with Wendy. There was definite concern but no explanation. Both women were just beside themselves.

Thankfully, some good news or at least encouraging news arrived soon after that scary ordeal with the state tests. Doctors from St. Vincent Mercy Medical Center told the Browns Alexa was eligible for the clinical study at the University of Vermont. The trial was focusing on a drug that had shown promise in the treatment of her type of cancer.

During this same time, the state of Ohio had announced that it had officially figured out that "something" (not sure what, but "something") caused the cancer in these kids. It was not just a "random cluster." And that was new. The defeatist attitude, however, was not. "When you take a look at studies like this across the country, rarely does anyone find the smoking gun," said Robert Indian in a late-May interview.

He did point out that his research indicated whatever had caused the cancer outbreak had since passed the area. It was no longer a threat.

To this day, I cannot figure out how they could have determined that especially when new cases were being added even when I was writing this book. I have asked, and the reason they gave was that "the number of cases had dropped since the height of the outbreak." However, children were still getting cancer. I know there can be a latency stage for cancers that can wildly vary in range of onset to diagnosis. However, the idea that it had all come and gone was not one that was acceptable to the many people who heard loved ones told they have cancer, or watched them die because of it.

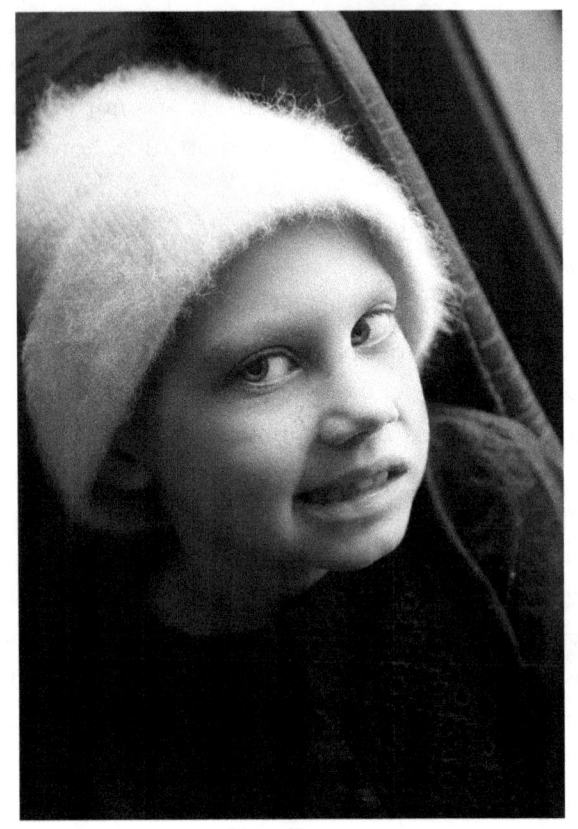

Alexa Brown

"We pray for you in church and on Wednesday evenings at Bible Study. God can do the things we can't do but hang on sweetie, lots of people love all of you."

Connie String from New Jersey
On CaringBridge.com

chapter 16

"News 11's investigation into a childhood cancer cluster in-and-around Clyde has led the way in getting more answers for the families involved," said anchor Jerry Anderson on an early June of 2009 11pm newscast. It was the start of my coverage entitled "Alexa's Journey."

Previously the Browns told me they were heading up to Vermont for the chance at a clinical trial. I knew I wanted to go with them to document everything. I also knew our station didn't have the budget to let me do that. So, I started thinking about what we could do to make sure we had enough information and pictures to share with the people of northwest Ohio. I remembered we had a handheld camera that the weather guys used when they went on school visits. I had to ask if we could use it.

"So, they are going to Vermont," I started telling Mitch Jacob while sitting in his office. Mitch had taken over a corner office that was originally used as a conference room. He was always very supportive of my coverage on the cancer cluster.

As soon as I was about to finish my sentence about the meteorologists' camera, Mitch did it for me. "Let's get them a camera to take with them," he blurted out. I smiled.

"That's a great idea," I answered. "I know we can't give them our regular news cameras, but what about the weather department's handheld camera?" I asked.

"Perfect. Make sure they have plenty of tapes and have them FedEx them back to us as they go through each day." Mitch's voice was excited. I was excited, too, but I knew I had to convince the family how important the taping was. They had to be committed to it even though it was not going to be pleasant.

I immediately left Mitch's office and walked quickly to my desk about 60 feet away. I snatched up my ugly, off-white phone with dirty push buttons and dialed Warren Brown.

"Warren? It's Jonathan. I have an idea that could really put a focus on Alexa's trip to Vermont," I told him while holding the phone to my ear and looking up on the internet how long it would take them to drive to the hospital up there. I then described what we wanted to do.

"Oh, Jonathan," Warren said. My heart sunk fearing that this request was perhaps too much. "I don't know," he continued. "I would have to talk to Wendy and the girls because I'm not even going. Wendy, Abby, Amanda and Alexa are all taking the trip and Ethan and I are staying back," he explained.

"Okay," I said without disappointment in my voice even though I was sensing his reluctance. I understood his hesitation. I also knew the importance of this kind of access to the family's struggles and the real-life video of exactly what it's like having a child with cancer. Or having it as a child. It was an unprecedented trial with an unorthodox coverage idea.

"Obviously, it's completely up to you, Warren. I have to tell you, though, if you want people to see what it's like to take care of a child with cancer and go through what could be a miracle treatment for Alexa, then this is the next best thing to having me and a photographer right there with you. In fact, it may be even better since the girls will just be themselves around each other rather than having us as an outside element trying to blend in with our big camera and microphone," I tried to explain. There was a long pause. I held the phone to my ear and stopped my internet search.

"I see what you're saying, Jonathan," Warren sighed. "I get it. I'll just have to convince Wendy this is what we need to do."

"I think it could be very powerful, Warren," I said with full conviction.

"I know it would be, Jonathan, but what if the trip doesn't work out?" he questioned.

It was one of the first times I heard Warren express a realization of what could very well be the final step in this experience. If she goes, gets the treatments, and they end up not being effective—that's going to be a lot of vulnerable emotion to document for everyone to see.

"Warren, we will only do what you're comfortable with," I reassured him. "You guys talk about it and let me know. We are ready to make it happen if you're okay with this," I told him as I leaned back into my chair and closed my eyes.

"I'll let you know. Thank you, Jonathan," Warren said in a deflated tone. I could tell he knew he would have to convince everyone this is the right thing to do if more attention was going to be paid to the problem of childhood cancer.

During that same time, Alexa got that "funny look" on her face again when talking to Sheryl Conley. On this occasion, it was all about the Vermont trip. Sheryl saw that look and braced herself for whatever was about to come out of Alexa's mouth.

"You know there's no reason for me to go," Alexa said to Sheryl.

Despite the preparation, Sheryl was kind of surprised. "What?" Sheryl asked.

"I don't need to go there," Alexa told her "grandmother."

Sheryl wanted to ask why Alexa felt that way, but instead kept it more positive. "Well, they might be able to help you. Maybe this will be the answer to our prayers," Sheryl said encouragingly.

Alexa just looked down, didn't say anything, and showed she really had no hope. However, in true Alexa style, she decided she needed to try.

Jerry Anderson reported that June night. "Tonight, we start a new chapter in this story giving you an even more up-close and personal look at how these cancer cases are affecting the families," he told our viewers. The family had said "yes" to my idea.

The first tapes came into the newsroom and were on my desk when I got into work about 3pm. I saw the envelope and knew exactly what they were. I barely dropped my workbag and still had my suit coat on a hanger in my hand when I reached for the package. I ripped it open and two mini-tapes popped out. I ran to the master control room where they took all the satellite feeds, ran the commercials, kept programming on the air, and taped various things for the newscasts.

The production staff dubbed off the video and I ran back to the edit bays to see just what they had captured.

"Say goodbye to everybody," I heard Amanda's voice say. She was in the backseat of the SUV with Amanda pointing the lens in Alexa's direction. Alexa did not seem happy about being taped. She sat staring straight ahead. Her head had just a little bit of hair and her smile was just as crooked as ever.

As I watched the video, Ethan leaned into the open window of the car and gave Alexa a kiss. Then, Warren came into frame and did the same thing telling Alexa he loved her. Then, in true family "vacation" video form, Amanda panned to the dogs that appeared to be saying goodbye as well. "There are the dogs, Lexa," she said as the good-sized canines jumped and barked. As soon as I saw this real family video, I knew this was exactly what people who have never had to deal with this needed to see. The Browns were just like any other family dealing with cancer. The disease attacks even the most normal of people.

That night on the air during the 5pm news, I described what we called the "nuts and bolts" of the story; the facts and logistics of what this story was all about.

"Alexa will be part of a Phase 2 trial of the drug Nifurtimox which was used for treating Chagas Disease and a sleeping sickness but also showed promise in cancer treatment," I told the viewers in the early newscast. "See more of Alexa's Journey tonight at 11," I said, tossing it back to the anchors.

As I walked out of the studio, I pulled my earpiece out and had my scripts in my hand. I looked up and saw Mitch near my desk. "Did you get some good stuff," he asked.

"Mitch, it's going to be powerful," I told him not knowing just how much impact this coverage would have here and across the globe.

As part of my introduction for the 11pm piece, I told the audience about how the family had been rolling tape during their trip, capturing candid moments. I started with that very first scene I watched on the raw tape.

"Wait. Look at me. Let's see those big eyes," said Amanda as she took the camera and focused it on Alexa. That stare I told you about was on display to begin my report of Day 1 of Alexa's Journey.

"All right, I'm going to zoom in on your freckles," teased Amanda as the camera honed in on the cute spots dotting the beautiful little girl's face. Alexa was having none of it. "Oh, Lex! The camera wants to see your freckles," Amanda explained but Alexa turned away. "Okay. Fine. I love you," she told her younger sister.

"Give your brother a kiss goodbye," Amanda told Alexa.

My voice then chimed in, "With a News 11 camera in hand, Alexa Brown's new video blog started this past weekend when she left her brother, dad and the dogs," I narrated.

"There's Alexa," Amanda said in her sweet, friendly voice. Alexa finally relented and gave a short wave to the camera. "Oh, I got a wave from her," Amanda said as she caught it all on tape.

During the report I described how the family was searching for a new treatment for Alexa's Medulloblastoma. It's a brain tumor that slowly steals the life out of young people that are supposed to be filled with life. The next shot on the tape showed Alexa asleep.

"There's Alexa sleeping again," explained Amanda on the tape.

I told the audience the past three years have been exhausting for Alexa…first a brain tumor and now cancer in her spine. It had gotten so bad that she had lost the use of her now tiny, thin, and undefined legs.

The home video showed how the sisters had to carry Alexa from the car to the bathroom at a rest stop along the way.

The trip had many ups and downs emotionally for the women and Alexa. They wanted to keep things on a positive note (as much as they could). When they stopped for the night near Rochester, NY, they visited at a Target store to pick up a new swimsuit for the young girl.

"What do you think, Channel 11?" the girls asked as they showed their options to the camera. It was a light moment of the day and a much-needed break for their minds. When dinner rolled around, the reality of Alexa's condition came flooding back. In the video, we saw Wendy toting around all of the medications she had to bring with her.

"Alexa's appetite has been really good since she's been on her steroid," explained Amanda while taping what was in her mom's medication bag. "She's on a steroid called Decadron for inflammation in her spine," announced Amanda in a sobering tone.

The video then showed the family a little later, with Alexa in her new bathing suit holding onto the railing in the hotel's hot tub.

"Whoo! Good job," said Amanda as she was taping Alexa and Abby in the water. Alexa showed off her arm strength by doing pull-ups on the railing. Then they explained more about her leg problems.

"Alexa's had some major trouble with her legs and has not been walking for at least a month," Abby explained as she sat in the tub right next to Alexa on the railing. "We're going to get her legs working again. Right, Alexa?" said Abby with no response from the little cancer patient.

"Say, 'Yes, I'm going to walk again'," coaxed Amanda.

"Yeah," Alexa said in a quiet and unconvincing voice. Alexa knew this was going to be an uphill battle.

At the end of each update on Alexa's Journey, we told our audience they could track the trip through our station's website and the CaringBridge.com journal that the family was keeping. Those sources would prove to be such a valuable asset for other families and children who were waging the same war on cancer.

Day two of our coverage included an early report in the 5pm news on how the family eventually checked in to the Ronald McDonald House in Burlington, Vermont. Plus, it showed just how taxing the whole experience had been on the family.

"Painful for Alexa especially—and for those of us who have to watch her go through it," described Abby on the home video tape. "But at times, it's been inspiring."

My 11 o'clock report had some of the family's brighter moments in it. "Amanda has her camera and she's taking a picture of me filming her," narrated Abby in the car as she was in the front seat looking at the back seat. Amanda has always loved still photography. At this point in the trip, Amanda gave the video camera to Abby and picked up her still camera to help document the trip from a different perspective.

Despite the moments of fun, I reminded the audience, "Don't

forget the seriousness of this desperate trip. They are all reminded of just what they're dealing with as they have to carry Alexa." Just as I'm saying that, the viewers saw the young ladies with Alexa in their arms as they walked down the halls of the Ronald McDonald House.

I go on to describe how they had to remember Alexa's medication after dinner one night.

"A steroid, a nerve medicine, and a narcotic," Wendy told the camera as we saw her in a restaurant booth looking down at her purse with bottles inside. "All because Alexa is having a lot of pain on a regular basis," the worried mom told the camera in a frustrated voice. She was not mad at Alexa. She was angry because as a mom she wants to protect her child, but not even the strongest of motherly love can heal the physical toll that cancer takes.

The report continued back inside the Ronald McDonald House with Amanda operating the camera again and asking her family to describe cancer in one word or phrase.

"What would it be?" Wendy contemplated. "Something that to us has become everyday life," she concluded.

"I would say painful," Abby said looking into the camera after it panned to her side of the room.

What about Alexa?

"Annoying," she said very sheepishly, staring down and away from the camera.

"That's fine," said Amanda. "That's an acceptable word to describe cancer," she added.

"How about stupid?" Alexa said.

"Thank you," said Amanda.

"Dumb," said Alexa.

"Dumb!" yelled Amanda to add emphasis on Alexa's timid voice.

No truer words were ever spoken by such a young girl as day three would ultimately prove.

The day at the Vermont Children's Hospital started in the wee hours of the morning with Alexa eating her favorite donut…chocolate. The long MRI process lasted hours that morning and afterward Alexa was worn out. Her sisters tried to cheer her up with gifts and cards.

"Three simple words," Alexa read and could be seen on video. "I love you. Love, Amanda," Alexa completed the card. Amanda planted a kiss on her baby sister.

During my reports on the trip, I showed how the women tried everything they could to take Alexa's mind off the cancer. But even their best efforts could not overshadow the realities.

"They just wanted to see animals on a farm," I told our viewers during my taped story. It was Shelburne Farms, a 1400-acre working farm complete with a forest. It's a National Historic Landmark.

"A definite long trek up a tough road with a wheelchair," I described but the pictures really told the story. The video showed a wide shot of a lengthy dirt path. Abby was desperately trying to push the wheelchair through the mud. Her battle with gravity did not help but that did not stop them from getting Alexa to see the animals.

"Obviously, you can see this is quite a steep hill to push a wheelchair up," narrated Amanda on the home video.

Even after that ordeal, the women would not quit. One of the locals told them it was "easy" to get to a scenic view of Lake Champlain. Maybe it was easy for able-bodied people, but the Brown's video showed a different story.

The women took turns carrying Alexa through the rough terrain and dragging the wheelchair alongside them. The rugged trip took nearly everything out of them by the time they reached the summit.

It was a breathtaking view of the hills and water. All of it while the women were out of breath from the hike. They took time to take some of it in, but the narration clearly showed how tired they were at that point.

"We just made it to the top of Mt. Everest," said Wendy. It just felt that way. "Here we are," she said looking over the water and the video captured a wide shot of the blue sky, dotted with white clouds and the calming waters below the green vegetated hills. The camera panned down to Amanda sitting on the ground, arms behind her propping her up, and looking like exhaustion had overtaken her face.

Alexa tried to help with the wheelchair every once in a while. In a parking lot, the video revealed Alexa's little arms hard at work.

"Here's Lexa pushing herself," Amanda said on tape. "She sometimes does this and does a pretty good job," she said proudly.

I reminded the audience that this was not easy. None of this was easy. It was easier when you a get a stuffed bear from the Vermont Teddy Bear Factory like they did during a side adventure on this trip. But it was not fun thinking about the next day's bone marrow aspiration and biopsy.

"I think there might be some tears and screaming," Amanda admitted on tape while back at the Ronald McDonald House that night. They knew tomorrow was not going to be fun, but once again, they did not have the clear vision of the kind of day it would be. It would take the family in yet another direction.

"Alexa is a sleepy little girl," said Amanda as she pointed the camera on her sister in bed. It was the start of a day that Alexa hoped would be THE DAY she started to really attack the cancer that had taken over her body.

"Here's the children's pediatric center," explained Amanda as we see Alexa being wheeled through the sliding glass doors of the facility. As excited as she was to get into the cancer trial, she still does not want to be there. The next shot showed Alexa all by herself in the wheelchair as it headed down a long hallway. The sunlight came pretty strongly through big windows, so Alexa appeared as a silhouette.

"This is Alexa escaping," Amanda said in a quiet voice standing back from the action. She got the shot of the little girl pushing herself. "She tends to do this. She hates when people follow her. She hates everything about cancer," Amanda said.

Despite the anesthesiologist performing some magic tricks for Alexa, there was no magic that could take away the excruciating pain of the procedure. Nor would there be magical news about Alexa's prospects of fighting her cancer.

Despite the MRI being done the two days earlier, no one had taken a look at the results before the excruciating bone marrow procedure. It would prove to be useless.

Just as Alexa was recovering from the procedure, the doctor called Wendy into an office. "You see these spots on the MRI?" asked the physician. There were numerous dark spots that dotted the brain. They were all over the place.

"Were they there before you came to see us?" the doctor questioned.

Wendy's face sunk. Her mind went numb. She could not believe her eyes as she scanned the dots on the sheet. Where did those come from? Wendy eventually answered the doctor's question. "No," she said in a hushed and stunned voice.

"I'm sorry, but Alexa can't go through the clinical trial," said the doctor. "With these new results, she doesn't fit the criteria anymore. There's nothing we can do," she added.

Wendy was still looking at the sheet. Her eyes eventually tilted up and made contact with the physician's eyes. It was a hollow feeling. Once again there's "nothing" they can do. The cancer was out of control and too aggressive.

Warren talked about the decisive blow on his blog. "Terrible news today. The Vermont MRI revealed new spots and a three-centimeter-long tumor in Alexa's brain. It must have been growing quite aggressively during the past four weeks because her brain area was stable after the last MRI at St. V's in Toledo."

Shortly after the devastating news, Alexa still wanted to make the most of the evening. the Browns stopped to visit a local book store and a Ben & Jerry's shop. Then it was back on the road to Ohio. The wheels were rolling and so was the camera again.

"We're on our way home because Lexa does not qualify for the study anymore," said Amanda with a noticeable, heavy heart. She was in the backseat again with Alexa. The camera was pointed at her sister whose face showed grave disappointment. "Unfortunately, the doctor can't help us," she added. "Hopefully, God will come through," she added on the verge of tears. The camera still showed the deadpan stare on Alexa's freckly face.

Once they were back in Clyde, Warren tried to take the news in stride. "We all know what's happening and we're dealing with it," he said on the tape. I asked the family to keep the camera to continue documenting what was going on with Alexa's Journey.

At Alexa's adamant request, just after hearing she did not qualify for the clinical trial, the family vowed to be upbeat by throwing a combined party for Ethan and Abby. Ethan had just passed his driver's test and got his license and it was Abby's birthday. What was interesting about Alexa was that even in her darkest hour when doctors told her she was not eligible for the Vermont study (that very day she heard those words) she was still thinking of others.

"Alexa went to the gift shop after all that bad news and she got me a birthday present," said Abby tearing up on the videotape. "It was very nice of her to think about me during that time," she continued.

Can you imagine a more mature, giving, selfless 11-year-old girl? She was basically told, "You're going to die." However, she did not wallow in that news. She bought her sister a birthday gift. I often think about that very moment as I deal with my own life challenges. I try to keep my focus on what I can do, not what has been said or done in the past. Alexa is and always was an amazing little girl.

Shortly after getting home, Amanda wrote on the CaringBridge.com blog. "I am asking God to send her a breath of fresh air that isn't poisoned by the word 'cancer.' She deserves to live without being scared. So, to everyone who reads this, continue to pray for help, strength, comfort and peace. Pray for a miracle."

At that same time, Sheryl Conley was helping her son clean up his condo. While she had a rag in her hand, she noticed her son's laptop on the table.

"Does that thing get on the internet, Tommy?" she asked wanting to check the progress of the Brown's trip to Vermont. She logged into CareBridge.com, read the posting from Amanda, and then collapsed on the floor in tears. "Oh, no!" she cried as Tommy and his wife ran over to comfort her.

It was no use. The sobbing was uncontrollable. Sheryl knew the end was near.

The Browns, though, continued to look for that miracle on earth through treatments and medicine. That same month had them off to more appointments.

"Where are we going?" Alexa asked in the car.

"To the hospital," answered Wendy as the video camera was rolling.

"To get what?" asked Alexa.

"Platelets," said Wendy in a here-we-go-again tone. Again, no one can blame her for her less-than-enthusiastic attitude.

"How are you feeling today?" asked the doctor once they were at their appointment.

"Fine," the little voice answered back.

"Your tummy hurt a little bit but that's because you had what? You swallowed like 25,000 pills," Wendy added.

Wendy had no quit in her whatsoever. She was now talking with a nutritional expert trying to start Alexa on a new protocol. As it was, the steroid she was on made her very hungry and Alexa gained a bit of a sweet tooth.

Through all of this, Alexa still had a sense of humor. She made her brother write a note one day. "I promise that I didn't steal or eat your peanut butter pie. Signed, Ethan Brown," read Alexa's brother while sitting in her bed with his younger sibling. He had a smile on his face and Alexa managed one of her patented crooked grins.

The news at the hospital was that her white blood cells were down. "That means Alexa can't be around anyone who is ill. So, if we see you and you have a cold, stay away from Alexa," Wendy told the camera.

The month of June wore on and the Browns were committed to making whatever time they had with Alexa the best it could be, despite her deteriorating health.

"We're hoping to have fun today at the zoo with my longtime, best friend Janet. We want to see the new baby elephant," said Wendy on her way to Columbus in late June. She was running the camera now. "Here's Alexa. She's taking her pills, eating a sandwich before we go to the zoo," Wendy narrated as the lens captured a quick meal.

It was a "normal" family day for the Browns. It was as normal as it could be with a child battling cancer and riding around in a wheelchair. Normal in the sense that they were taking pictures of all the monkeys, leopards, and fish, catching a ride on the merry-go-round (although, Alexa had to be held up on the horse), and enjoying the sunny day.

At one point near the gorilla cage, Amanda was taping Alexa in her wheelchair looking at the exhibit. Amanda had been trying to get

Alexa to talk to the camera about her trip to the zoo, but to no avail.

"All right," said Amanda.

"All right," said Alexa.

"All right," said Amanda again.

"All right," said Alexa again but this time with a crooked smirk.

"Stop mimicking me," Amanda shouted with a chuckle.

"Stop mimicking me," laughed Alexa.

"Can you wave to me," asked Amanda. Alexa complied.

"Thank you," Amanda said.

There was still a typical little sister in that cancer-ridden body…a little sister who loved her family and loved teasing her siblings just the same, like any other "normal" family.

The videotape captured moments of smiles, waves, and laughs. At the end of the day, it was a good experience to remember, but a long day for the unhealthy girl.

The next few days of taping showed Alexa enjoying some ice cream and talking about going shopping. Alexa was losing more of her hair again although she was not receiving more treatments. The family was trying to keep her busy, trying to keep her mind off what was happening.

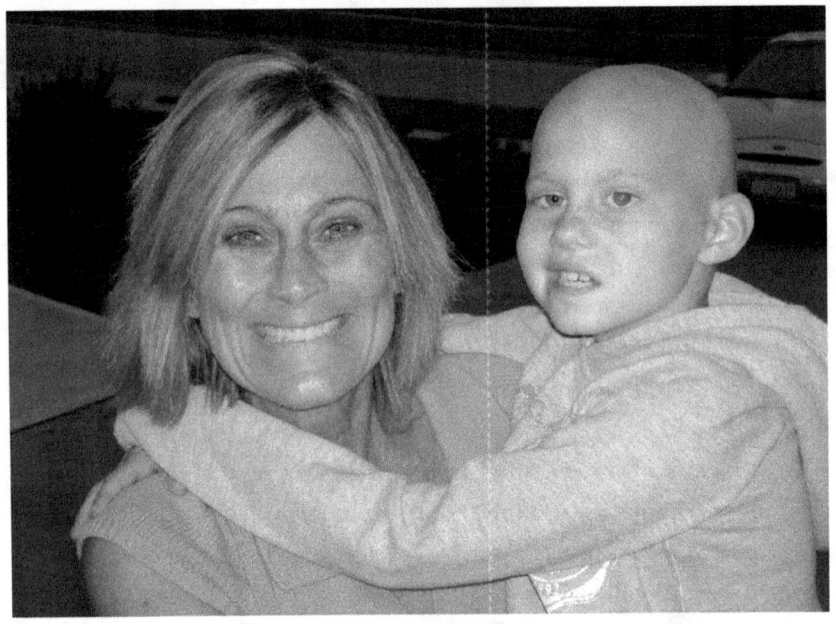

Wendy Brown, Alexa Brown

"I don't know if you remember us, we live in Morocco! I went to high school and college with your Mom and to college with your Dad. I'm from Clyde and my wife is from Pennsylvania. We're praying for you and hope you get well soon!"

Steve and Betsy from Morocco
On CaringBridge.com

chapter 17

One day Amanda picked up the camera and taped what had become a very special time for Alexa every chance she got.

"Alexa is examining some letters she recently received from a church in Bellevue," she explained as the camera showed numerous letters all over the bed she was in. It was not just mail from Ohio. There were hand-written notes from across the country. Alexa was reaching thousands of people. This little girl in this big battle from a small town was making a huge impact through the CaringBridge.com journal and the news coverage of her journey.

"What a beautiful name," read Alexa. "My name is Jennifer and I live in New York City," she continued. As she read the many letters, Amanda took a moment to interrupt and explain what the family's next steps for the little girl would be.

"We've been in touch with a doctor from California," said the big sister. "Hopefully they'll come up with a new treatment scheme for Lexa. We're still praying for a miracle and we believe God will give us one," she said in an upbeat voice. "Many, many people prayed on that cloth," she went on to explain as she panned to a piece of material that appeared to be a "healing cloth."

"So, we have it with her at all times even when she's sleeping," Amanda recorded on tape.

"And my mom puts it on my head," said Alexa.

That was taped toward the end of June. Even in the most desperate stage of this fight, it was a special time for a promise made by Sheryl Conley. Sheryl's sister owned a horse named Kibby; a horse that Alexa always wanted to ride. There were so many times they tried to make the arrangements for Alexa to get on that horse but something inevitably would come up.

Sheryl's sister would be out of town, or it didn't fit into Alexa's hospital treatment schedule, or Sheryl had to be with her sons. They finally came up with a date that seemed to work but then there was a phone call.

"You can't come over," said Sheryl's sister. "They're cutting the timothy hay," she explained. Sheryl has a bad case of asthma and every time there was a thick portion of timothy hay in the air, Sheryl had to go indoors and close the windows. Otherwise, she would have to be admitted to the hospital. It was that bad.

Sheryl was not about to put this ride off for yet another minute, so her sister agreed that Amanda and Alexa could go. Sheryl called the Brown's home to tell Alexa the exciting news.

"I'm not going to be able to go today, but you and Amanda can go and…" said Sheryl but her sentence was quickly interrupted.

"I'm not going if you're not going," Alexa shouted back as she broke out into tears. Alexa couldn't even talk; she was so upset. She put down the phone and Amanda picked it up. Sheryl had to think quickly, again. Alexa seemed to pull that weaker skill out of Sheryl.

"Get Alexa again," Sheryl told Amanda. The crying little "granddaughter" put the phone back to her ear.

"You didn't listen to me all the way," said Sheryl. "You're not going to ride Kibby today. You're going to meet Kibby today so the next time when we go out together, then the horse will know you and you can ride her. That way the timothy hay won't have just been cut, I'll be there with you, and I won't miss seeing you ride her." Alexa bought it. Sheryl wiped her worried, line-filled, sweating brow.

When Alexa got to the farm, she met that horse…big, brown and white, beautiful. There was no way Alexa was leaving that day without getting on the animal. Amanda and Sheryl's sister made it happen.

When they were done that day, Alexa and Amanda went to Sheryl's house before heading home. Alexa was so excited she could barely get all the words out quickly enough to tell Sheryl about the experience.

"And then I fed her and she really liked the food I had…and then she bent her nose down so I could pet it and she was really, really soft… and then I petted her side…and then I got up on her…and then…, and then…, and then…" Alexa rolled on and on, showing Sheryl the pictures that captured the magical day. There was nothing but smiles and laughter that filled that room.

Toward the end of that visit, Alexa told Sheryl she wanted to bake later that week. She told Sheryl that Amanda could come, too.

"Oh, you can have some time alone with Sheryl," said Amanda in such a sweet, understanding voice. "It's okay," she added.

However, Alexa was insistent.

Later she would whisper in Sheryl's ear, "I don't think you can carry me."

Alexa's legs were not working at all at that point. She was just looking out for Sheryl…again.

"What kind of cookies do you want to bake?" asked Sheryl as the girls were getting their things together to leave for home.

"Have you used that new brownie pan yet?" asked Alexa.

"No," replied Sheryl.

"Then let's do brownies," said the child.

"I don't know where the pan is," said Sheryl.

"Well then find it," Alexa told "grandma." "You have the whole day," she finished.

Sheryl just smiled. That was Alexa.

Sure enough, the girls all got together. Alexa was determined to do the mixing of the batter. Warren was out in the front yard working on cutting up Sheryl's tree that had blown over in a storm earlier in the week. As he was hauling away the various pieces of wood, Amanda noticed her dad's hard work. She decided she should help him finish. She went outside and left Alexa and Sheryl alone.

"Would you do me a favor?" asked Alexa, seizing the moment of alone time.

"Sure," said Sheryl, although, she had seen that look on Alexa's face before.

"Will you make sure that Amanda makes it back to school?" asked the little girl.

"I can't do that, sweetie," said Sheryl. "I am not her parent. I have no control over her and I can't tell her what to do," she added.

"You have to, Sheryl. You have to make sure she goes back to school," pleaded the concerned sister.

That night they baked the brownies. Alexa then started to get tired. They had not decorated them yet, so Sheryl sent all of the decorations home with the Browns…icing, sprinkles, and those pesky M&M's. Alexa did manage to put an "S" on one brownie for Sheryl and a "T" on another for her husband Tom. It would be the last brownie-making session at Sheryl's home. They did not know that at the time. The whole event was savored and appreciated.

The next day proved to carry a very different tone. It was all shown on the home video camera.

"She did not sleep all night last night," Warren said as he sat on the front porch of their home. His attitude was dark and there was a reason for that.

"She awakened to find nothing but pain in her head and in her temples, in her legs and in her back," he struggled to let the camera know. "She writhed in pain all night long until about 15 minutes ago," he explained with a harsh, worried look on his face. Wendy took Alexa back to the hospital. This was the beginning of the end. Warren was fuming on the front porch.

"For those of you who listen to this tape and listen to me spout off for the next few minutes about how unjustly children with cancer have been treated in this country, I hope you'll take it to heart.

"What I'd like is for our representatives to get off your duffs in Washington and come sit on this porch in Clyde, Ohio and come speak to me man-to-man and face-to-face and tell me why it is that this child along with lots of other children in this country have to suffer in such a way," he said with a pounding of his fist every so often on the wooden armrest of his chair.

Warren went on to question why the United States was bailing out big companies and not worrying about our future generations that will continue to have to deal with cancer.

"Mr. Obama, take a look at pediatric cancer. I'm sure that if Alexa's last name was the same as yours, the floodgates of funding would fly open instantaneously," Warren said in his continued serious tone. It was not the first time (nor would it be the last time) Warren had a political tone to his thoughts on cancer. In fact, one high-ranking leader would eventually take him up on his "front porch summit" proposal.

For the time being, though, the attention needed to be given to Alexa. During the two-day hospital stay over the 4th of July, Alexa appeared to have suffered a stroke, but she held on. The Browns wanted to get her back home and comfortable. Her loved ones felt the end was very near. They asked two hospice nurses to come to the home and help take care of the little girl. The cancer was acting more aggressively and Alexa's fight to become that "normal" little girl was fading.

The harsh reality of how cancer affects families was rearing its ugly head and all of it was caught on tape. Despite how difficult it was for the family to sit beside and watch their beautifully spirited and gorgeous girl fade, the mission to draw attention to the problem of childhood cancer was not going to escape the lens of that camera we had given to the Browns.

Often it was Warren who picked up the camera and showed how the family was sitting in Alexa's bed, how friends were stopping by to give her a kiss, how much each person was crying because they could see the situation was getting direr by the second.

Alexa looked calm with her bald head and wearing her favorite purple pajamas. She was not responding. She was there in the room, but she wasn't there.

The video was difficult to watch, but give Warren credit for having the courage to tape the family's darkest of days. This was the true-life scenario thousands of families face every day, but the every-day "normal" families do not get to see what the cancer experience is really like. Warren and the family wanted everyone to take in the terribleness that is childhood cancer…to take in the pain, the emotion, the certain finality that many versions of this disease bring forth.

If you struggled to watch, it meant you understood. If you did not feel a thing while witnessing this little girl slowly slip away, you never would get the point of this "Journey." It was a chance Warren and the family were willing to take not just then but as you'll see, in the future, too.

You could see on the tape friends stopping by. Sheryl Conley was one of those supporters. But she didn't just visit every once in a while. She was there day in and day out. When she heard about Alexa's turn for the worse, Sheryl went into "fixing food mode" as she liked to call it and scheduled others to bring food, too. People made everything from lasagna to salads, to scrambled eggs and blueberry muffins. A lot of it was to help ease the family's worry about meals, but it was more about keeping her own mind off losing her special friend.

"Seeing her in that bed was worse than the time I saw her when she came home from the initial surgery and she was lying in the big chair," said Sheryl reflecting on that awful time. "There was at least hope when she came home from the hospital then, but when she came back this time, they told us there was such a short amount of time. She was brought home to die."

Knowing that time was limited, Sheryl got all the meals ready for the family who were in that bedroom constantly. When dinner was ready, though, they all came out to eat together. That provided Sheryl some time to spend with Alexa.

Sometimes she would read Winnie The Pooh and sometimes she just talked to Alexa. As she did, she held the little girl's hand. Alexa used that handholding as a way to communicate.

"I noticed a book in the room called 90 Minutes in Heaven," recalled Sheryl.

The book described an experience Don Piper had when he died in a car crash. He believed he went to Heaven.

"Would you like to know what Heaven's like?" asked Sheryl. Alexa squeezed Sheryl's hand. That meant yes.

"...a light enveloped me, with a brilliance beyond earthly comprehension or description," read Sheryl from the book. "In my next moment of awareness, I was standing in Heaven. Joy pulsated through me as I looked around, and at that moment, I became aware of a large crowd of people. They stood in front of a brilliant, ornate gate. I have no idea how far away they were; such things as distance didn't matter. As the crowd rushed toward me, I didn't see Jesus, but I did see people I had known. As they surged toward me, I knew instantly that all of them had died during my lifetime. Their presence seemed absolutely natural.

"They rushed toward me, and every person was smiling, shouting, and praising God. Although no one said so, intuitively I knew they were my celestial welcoming committee. It was as if they had all gathered just outside Heaven's gate, waiting for me," Sheryl's lips kept reading. "Everything I experienced was like a first-class buffet for the senses. I had never felt such powerful embraces or feasted my eyes on such beauty. Heaven's light and texture defy earthly eyes or explanation. Warm, radiant light engulfed me. As I looked around, I could hardly grasp the vivid, dazzling colors. Every hue and tone surpassed anything I had ever seen," wrote authors Don Piper and Cecil Murphey with their words now pouring out of Sheryl's mouth. Alexa had listened intently.

A couple days later Sheryl suggested a Whinnie the Pooh book but Alexa did not squeeze her hand.

"Something else?" asked Sheryl.

Squeeze.

Sheryl thought for a moment.

"You want to hear about Heaven again?" she questioned.

Squeeze.

The thoughts of dying did not agitate her. She was really interested in hearing more about Heaven. As Sheryl grabbed the book again, she remembered the question Alexa posed to her many months ago. "Are you afraid of dying?"

As Sheryl voiced the poignant words of the authors, she noticed Alexa's eyes changed and Alexa actually turned her head toward Sheryl's voice to listen to each description. That little turn of the head was hard for her to do. The pain was immense, but in Alexa's mind it was all worth it.

"My time with Alexa was life-changing for sure," reflected Sheryl. My experience all started with 'I don't want to do this' but ended with 'I'm so glad to be a part of her life.' I think I ended up learning more from her than she did from me." Those precious moments were some of the last Sheryl would have with Alexa. None of those moments were caught on the camera we provided, but all are deeply embedded in Sheryl's memory.

"We are just going hour-by-hour and day-by-day, waiting to see what occurs in her life," Warren said, continuing on that tape as he revisited the front porch for his time to vent. "Unfortunately, that's the commentary on federal funding for kids with cancer. Kids have no power. They have no say. They get nothing," Warren said staring down the camera as if to look into the soul of the legislators. "We need more help...not just for my child because, quite frankly, there's nothing that can be done for my child, but for the possibility to squash childhood cancer," he added with a stern look.

After Alexa returned from Vermont and was falling tighter into cancer's evil embrace, the Ohio EPA announced it was doing water testing. Reps collected samples from Clyde's Beaver Creek Reservoir. "The Ohio EPA thought it was a good idea to do some additional testing to see if it could be of any help in the investigation," said one of the researchers.

They were looking for any chemicals that may have played a role in the childhood cancer cluster. "The extra testing we'll be doing is for pesticide compounds. One of those is DDT which is a compound that has been banned for quite a few years," he explained. We came to find out that many of the compounds they were looking for can stay in the environment for years after they are used. The Beaver Creek Reservoir was especially important because it was the drinking water supply for people in Clyde.

"I'm very glad that they're continuing the testing," said Ned McElfresh during one of our interviews on the testing. He was a life-long resident of Clyde who had two children of his own. The need for answers went deeper than just his own family, though. "We have some friends of the family where both their daughter and their son are part of that cluster, so we'd like to see something resolved," he said referring to the Hisey family. The reps went on to say that the Ohio EPA would be testing other bodies of water in the Clyde area to add what they could to the investigation.

On a federal level, I was contacting house representatives and senators, informing them about the devastating mystery that plagued these tiny towns. Some had never heard of the situation before, like Senator Sherrod Brown's office. No relation, by the way, to Warren and Wendy Brown.

As I dialed the senator's office, I was transferred to his press secretary. I remember sitting at my little desk in Toledo, OH thinking if these people don't know about this cancer cluster after years of reporting, I would be very surprised. They did not know about it, but much to Senator Brown's credit, his office did not pretend to know. As I told them the long details and sent them numerous reports I had done in the past, they were all very receptive and thankful that I had called their attention to such a horrible situation. They told me they would be in contact with the family soon. I hung up the phone and felt the info I just gave could very well be a turning point for the amount of attention this case would get. I would soon know that I was correct.

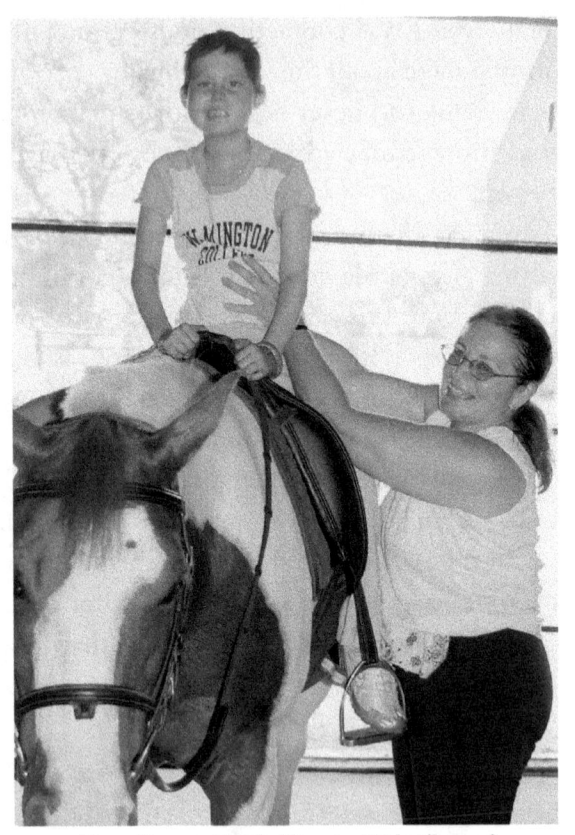

Alexa Brown, Karrie Flower, Kibby (horse)

"Alexa, you are one of the strongest people I know. That's not just talking about kids, adults, too. Your strength in the face of struggle is an inspiration to so many people. You are well loved and cherished for who you are and who you help us to be."

Jonathan

chapter 18

"Hey, Jonathan, can you help us out?" asked Warren during a late-June conversation.

"Whatcha' need, my friend?" I asked as I was driving around in our worn-out news vehicle and talking on an overworked cell phone.

"The town is throwing a big event for the 4th of July and we need someone to emcee our 'Clyde's Got Talent' show. It'll be held at the park and then there will be fireworks that night. Wendy and I would like to invite your family over to the house for a cookout after the show and then we can see the fireworks from our house," Warren explained.

I thought it was a great idea. My family always heard so much about the Browns and saw the many reports I had done about Alexa, but they had not yet met them in person.

"Count us in," I told him with a smile. "My kids will love hanging out and watching the fireworks," I added.

"Oh yeah. It's one of Alexa's favorite things, too. She loves fireworks," Warren said, laughing a bit. "OK, Jonathan, thank you. I look forward to spending some time together outside of all the news coverage," Warren said with a sigh.

"Yeah. Me, too. Can't wait," I told him.

My family and I never made it to the Browns for food and fun. That conversation happened just before Alexa had taken a final turn downward in what had always been a valiant fight.

Warren's invitation took place just days before Warren would tape a well-deserved rant on his front porch about Washington D.C., lawmakers, and the unfair system of healthcare for children. When he and I laughed about the fireworks over the phone, it was the last time I would personally hear Warren laugh for quite a while.

Warren kept rolling with the videotape inside the home, until the bitter end. Tears flowing from every family member, each of them exhausted, each not giving up a spot right next to Alexa in bed.

One time, in a state of punchiness, the sisters in their tired bodies found a second wind as they pulled out some CDs. The video showed the only light moments the family had in late July and early August. "Umm Bop…do…do…doo bop." The music blared and the sisters' singing just barely overpowered the ridiculous song from the group "Hanson." The boy band had three brothers. The Browns had three sisters.

Alexa was unable to sing but could no doubt hear the bouncing lyrics booming from her siblings. Those two older sisters could move and dance. The once very athletic, coordinated 11-year-old girl who had been so active could only sit up in bed motionless. The girls were trying anything they could to help Alexa, to encourage their sister, and to give her something else to think about besides cancer.

In those weeks of late July and into early August, I was getting updates from the family and their on-line journal entries. The tone of the writing was not confident about Alexa being able to bounce back from this latest cancer attack.

On August 6, 2009, I got a phone call at home.

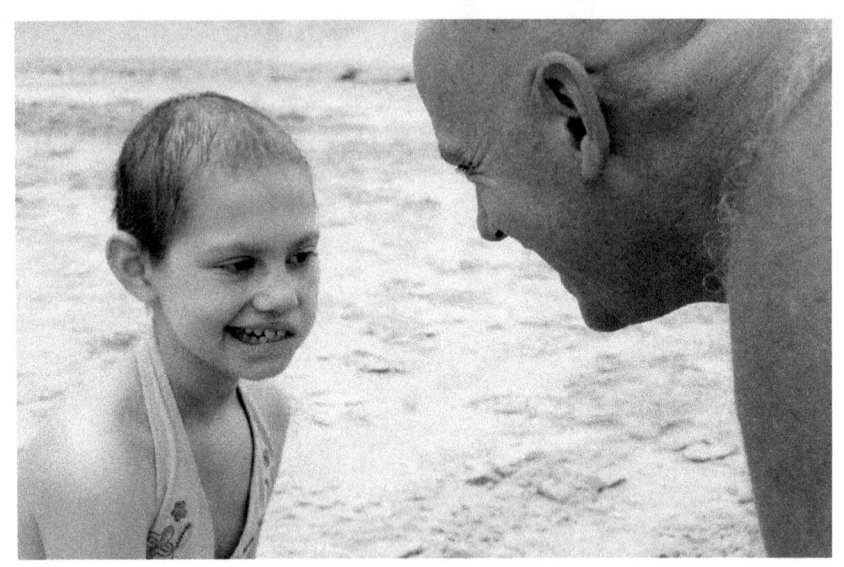

Alexa Brown, Warren Brown

"One-year anniversary and many tears have been shed and many more to come before this day is over. Between the moments of tearfulness, Alexa's message of hope and determination in the face of unbeatable odds does and will continue to resonate within each of us."

Warren
On CaringBridge.com

chapter 19

I worked the night shift and I worked weekends. It was a Thursday morning. Thursdays were normally my day off. I had just woken up around 9am.

"Jonathan, it's Andi," said my new news director, Andi Roman. She took over for Mitch Jacob, who left for a job in Columbus. His departure came during the middle of Alexa's downturn in health.

"Hey, Andi. What's happening?" I asked with a pep to my voice although I knew that when I got a call from the news director on my day off, it was generally not good news. My fear came to fruition.

"Did you hear?" she asked softly.

"Hear what?" I said.

"Jonathan, I'm so sorry but the Browns just wrote that Alexa passed away this morning."

Dead silence. My heart sank. It broke. I started to cry. It was the first time I had cried in many, many years.

I held the cordless phone to my ear saying nothing but my mind was racing. Why? Why did she have to die? How are the Browns doing? I have to get ahold of them. Do they want to hear from me right now? How do we handle this news? What are the funeral arrangements? Andi finally broke the silence.

"Take some time to think about what you want to do," Andi said. She's a mother. In this situation, I was so glad to have that compassion. "Give me a call back when you can," she told me.

"Thank you, Andi," I said with a cracking voice.

I hung up the phone. I sat down at my kitchen table with my head in my hands and still wearing what I had gone to bed in last night.

"She's better off," I said to myself. No more pain.

"Why the hell did this happen?" I raged at times.

It was a good half-hour before I finally knew what I had to do.

As the buttons made their tones on the phone, I wondered what I was going to say. I had no idea. Warren picked up.

"Hello," his weak voice mumbled through the phone.

"Warren, I am so sorry," I said trying unsuccessfully to sound strong. I held it together but tears were streaming down my face.

"Jonathan, she's gone," Warren said breaking down.

"I know. I know," I told him trying to comfort the grieving father. How was there any comfort to give after what he and his family had been through? I tried. "She's not suffering anymore, Warren. The pain is gone," I told him fighting through additional tears.

"You're right, Jonathan. You're right," he said. There was a long pause in the conversation where all I heard through that stupid phone was sniffling. By this time, I was pacing my kitchen floor searching my mind for the right words, but not finding any of them appropriate. Feeling helpless, I then broke the near silence.

"Warren, I am sorry I didn't…if I had only…" I tried to say and Warren immediately interrupted knowing where I was about to go.

"No! No, Jonathan! Don't do that," he said in a firm tone all while still letting the raw emotion through. It made my tears flow even more hearing his pain.

"You did all you could to let people know about this," he told me. Somehow it felt like he was comforting me. Me? He just lost his daughter and he was worried about me. I am telling you. I have never met a family like this one. I have never met a more determined man like Warren Brown.

"That's why we have to talk to you today!" Warren told me without hesitation. At first, I was kind of taken aback, but then again, this was Warren. I should have expected it.

"I'll get into work early and be over to the house by two o'clock," I told him.

"OK, Jonathan. We'll see you then," Warren said.

"Warren, I'm sorry."

"Bye, Jonathan."

As I hung up the phone, I looked around the house. No one was there. The kids were at camp. My wife was out meeting a new business client. I was alone.

I sat back down at the kitchen table and wiped away the long trails of tears along my cheeks. It was over, but it had also just begun.

As I got ready for work, I turned on the noon news on WTOL.

"Some sad news this morning on 11-year-old Alexa Brown's Journey that News 11 has been closely following," said anchor Melissa Voetsch. "According to her family's journal, Alexa passed away at four o'clock this morning," she continued as video came up on the screen of the little girl lying in her bed at home.

They were pictures I had seen a thousand times, but this time they stopped me dead in my tracks. I looked at them. I stared at her little bald head and thought about the countless kisses from family and friends given on that beautiful head.

"Alexa's family posted on her journal, 'We can all rest easy knowing that Alexa will forever be protected by Jesus and a host of family members that have gone on before us.'"

I thought to myself, how true that is. So many of our friends and relatives have taken a journey to the other side. However, Alexa's journey was so different—so undeserved, and had ended way too soon.

"Her father Warren says Alexa was full of love and life," continued Melissa delivering the story. "And that today, she earned her angel's wings."

I turned away from the TV and continued getting ready. I had no idea how I was going to approach this interview.

After I got to work and hopped in our live truck. The ride with my photographer Shawn Dunagan was silent for the most part. Both of us knew the finality of what had happened that morning, but we also knew we had a job to do to further this "story."

"How do you want to handle this?" asked my young photographer. He had often looked to me for answers about what direction we should take the report that we were about to put together. Shawn had a respect for me and vice versa that did not need to be talked about. It was there. I knew he thought I had a plan for every scenario we would encounter…fires, crimes, features. This time, I was blank.

"To be honest with you, Shawny, I'm not really sure," I told him while sifting through dozens of past Alexa reports I had printed out just before we rolled down the highway. "I'm really not sure," I sighed. Shawn did not say a word.

We pulled our overbearing, News 11 truck through the tiny town and up to the Brown's cul de sac. The house looked quiet. Our truck was silent as we parked, shut off the engine and sat for a second staring at the home. I took a deep breath and the creaking of the old, rusty door made a screeching slice through the air.

We walked up slowly with our TV gear in hand. Wendy saw us approach.

"I'm sorry, Wendy," I said as she opened the door. I immediately gave her a hug. I hadn't talked to her yet. Her eyes were even more tired looking than ever before.

"Warren's getting his shirt on," said Wendy wiping away what must have been her ten-thousandth tear of the day. "I thought we could talk on the porch," she told us. "We'll be out in a minute."

We set up the camera and tripod. There were two oversized, wooden rocking chairs next to each other in front of me. I thought to myself how many times did they sit in these chairs before and think of the next steps for Alexa, planned their next day at the hospital for her treatments, and prayed that she would be whole again on earth? I can only imagine.

The Browns stepped out of the house and Warren gave me a big hug. I had no idea what to say. What do you say? No…really, what do you say?

"If you're not ready to do this, I completely understand," I blurted out. Not sure why I said that, because I knew Warren wanted to tell everyone how much all of this is flat out terrible. How we all need to know how devastating this day has already been.

"We need to do this, Jonathan," Warren told me as he took a seat. Wendy didn't say a word…probably still in shock, maybe even remembering the times she had sat in those rocking chairs thinking about her daughter.

"We're rolling," said Shawn in a quiet voice.

I had nothing planned. I just started asking whatever came to my mind.

"I know this is a dumb question right now, but how are you doing?" I asked.

"Uh, I'm doing all right for just having a daughter who died," said Warren. "Just because we knew that if God did not heal her here, she could no longer live how she had been living. So, now we know she's healed. She's fine. She's better off than we are," Warren said as his profound words pierced the air.

"Alexa had been suffering for a while," I pointed out. "Was there a time that you began preparing for this day?"

"If you give me a pair of pliers and a bale of wire and twine," Warren said with tears welling up. "I can pretty much fix everything, but I couldn't fix my daughter," he said. "I did come to grips with that, but nothing truly prepares you for the shock of losing a child," he told us.

"If she couldn't be healed here," Wendy said breaking her silence. "Then she had to be healed in Heaven," she continued with brief pauses and a trembling lower lip. The tears followed.

Warren told the camera that during her last days, he thought he had cried himself out. He could not have been more wrong.

"This morning as I was reaching under her head and reaching under her legs...I hate to be cliché but it hit me like a ton of bricks," Warren said while describing what he had to do when the funeral home staff arrived at the house. "I couldn't catch my breath," he sighed as he looked down shaking his head.

"We didn't want the stretcher coming into our home," Wendy said picking up the story. "So...we wrapped her up in her little Tinker Bell blanket," she continued with the tears too much for her to hold back. She paused, and then her weak voice said, "And he carried her out."

Warren wanted to carry his daughter. Her lifeless body wrapped in a colorful blanket was draped over his arms. The strength Warren had left in his tired muscles barely moved his weakened legs after such a long journey with cancer. What was normally a short walk seemed impossible. His slow steps took Alexa and him out the same front door that Alexa had come through every day after school. He struggled across the very porch where she had jumped rope so many times and through the green grass that Alexa had done too-many-to-count perfect cartwheels on. Warren shuffled slowly across the sidewalk where she had ridden her bicycle letting the breeze whip through her sandy blonde hair, and to the paved portion of the cul de sac where her roller blades had become familiar with every crack and seam. Warren placed his daughter into the waiting hearse.

"No parent should ever have to do that," Warren said to me during the interview. "No parent should ever have to carry a deceased child to the back of a waiting funeral car," he told me. He could not have been more right.

The hearse then drove off with his little girl. All he could do was stand and watch the wheels spin into a blur as the vehicle roll away from him—his youngest child inside.

"It didn't really hit me again until I walked back into the bedroom and I could smell her. They had been using a certain type of lotion," he told us as more tears came flooding through his words. "I could just smell her in our bed room where she'd been staying," he said fighting through the never-ending streams of pain leaving thick trails along his cheeks.

The saddened parents were quiet for a moment. I looked at them with their heads down. I asked them about who Alexa was.

"She was just a happy little girl who loved life," said Wendy who continued about her youngest child's accomplishments. She also shared Alexa's grounded, mature nature even through the worst kind of physical pains that cancer gave.

"I remember when she would be awake at night sometimes and couldn't sleep," recalled Wendy. "She'd say, 'Mom, you just go to sleep. I don't want to keep you up.' She did not want to be a burden to anybody," Wendy said with a far-off look in her eyes as if she was reliving those moments right there and then

"In fact, Jonathan," Warren popped in. "On the night of July 3rd, just before you and your family were supposed to join us, she was in so much pain. Her head was hurting. Then she had a spell when it didn't hurt quite as badly. She turned to her mom and pulled her mom down and said, 'I'm sorry you have to go through this with me. I wish I could be a normal kid. I wish I could live a normal life,'" Warren said with so much emotion in his voice. "That was the heart of Alexa Brown," the proud father told us with so much conviction that I could tell the tone of the interview was about to turn.

"As tough as this is to talk about, I'm not angry about…how she was. I am angry that she had to get cancer however it appeared in her body," said Warren. "I'm angry about whatever caused it here in Clyde. I'm angry there isn't enough research to get rid of it," he told us staring straight into the camera.

"Something has got to give," continued Warren. "We're going to get national attention. Somehow, some way we're going to get this the attention it deserves. Parents shouldn't have to deal with this," the father said as the rocking chair came to a standstill. He was in full motivation mode now. The tears were dry and a determined look came across the very face that just moments ago described the agony of carrying his deceased daughter.

"Today, as we speak, 40,000 families in the United States are affected by childhood cancer," Warren told us. "About 4,000 kids just like Alexa die each year. The reason it hasn't gotten any attention is because parents are caught in the middle of the fight and in the thick of it, battling for their child. They are either fighting with God to make their child whole or they're fighting with the medical community as to the next step. You can't advocate for yourself. There's no time. Kids get lost in this political mess, too. Kids can't get on the phone and dial Washington. They can't hop on a plane and go sit in the middle of the rotunda and yell, 'Here I am! I'm bald! Help me!' They don't have any power. So, it has to be somebody who can pick up the torch and keep it moving," Warren said with a straightened posture in the curved wooden seat.

Warren then told us how just a few days before Alexa had passed, a representative from U.S. Senator Sherrod Brown's office had visited their home and met Alexa. The Browns from little old Clyde had reached the Browns of big Washington, D.C.

"We've been successful with the help of WTOL, our media friends, and our partners through all of this. We put enough pressure on D.C. to actually have Sherrod Brown wanting to come to our porch to discuss this issue of childhood cancer and the need for additional funding for research," Warren said. My phone call informing the senator and his staff, plus the continued push from the Clyde Browns had finally made an impact.

"What will you ask him?" I asked Warren.

"How the disparity in funding between childhood cancer and adult cancer can be so apparent and not be addressed," Warren revealed to us. "It doesn't make any sense. That's what we're going to talk about. I told Alexa before she died that I will not rest until we get childhood cancer the attention it deserves. I already miss her," he said as his tougher tone cracked a bit. But he stiffened back up and stared back into the camera. "She's in Heaven. She's fine. Now we have to start concentrating on what we can do so this does not happen to other countless children," he added.

Remember, these parents had just lost their daughter a few hours ago.

We wrapped up the interview. I gave them some hugs and reassured them of my commitment. "I'll be there through all of this," I told them.

"I know you will, Jonathan. I know you will," Warren told me.

Later that afternoon, as I stood in the middle of the small downtown of Clyde, I figured out what I was going to say when the camera would be on. I wrote down the experiences of the day for the Brown family so I could inform our audience not only about how tragic this was, but also about the fight this family still had…even on that day. A day they never wanted to see.

"Her family plans to continue the fight against childhood cancer in her memory, Jonathan," said our anchor, Chrys Peterson…a mom herself, and someone who was deeply concerned about these cases. She was the chairperson of the Northwest Ohio Komen Race for the Cure that brings thousands of people to downtown Toledo every fall with one goal in mind—kick the crap out of cancer.

As she threw to me live in the field, whatever I prepared to say off the bat did not come out. It was as if something overtook me. I don't know how to quite explain it. That feeling has never happened to me before a live report. It was as if an outside influence stepped in. Where I had planned to be more matter-of-fact, I went into a deeper, introspective thought.

"Chrys, this family is unlike any I've met. Their strength amazes me," I just started reacting from my heart. That was not something we were really supposed to do as journalists, but as I was saying the words, I felt they were wholly appropriate at that time. "Who knows why Alexa had to go through this? Who knows why any of these children have to go through these cases of cancer…and some have to die. No one knows and that's the frustrating thing for these families, the Browns, this community and for me, too," I said not thinking but just talking.

I eventually did report about how Alexa died and how Warren had to carry his daughter out of the house. I also talked about the planned meeting with Senator Sherrod Brown. "Hopefully, Alexa's journey will have some impact on Washington," I said concluding the live shot.

"A memorial service is planned for next Saturday," said Chrys in the studio before concluding that night's coverage.

It was a day our staff will never forget. Chrys was heartbroken. My sturdy, keep-the-ship-going News Desk Manager Frank Seeley, who normally had a joke for any situation, was noticeably quiet only saying, "I'm sorry, Jonathan."

It was a somber newsroom as if we had lost someone very dear to us…because we had.

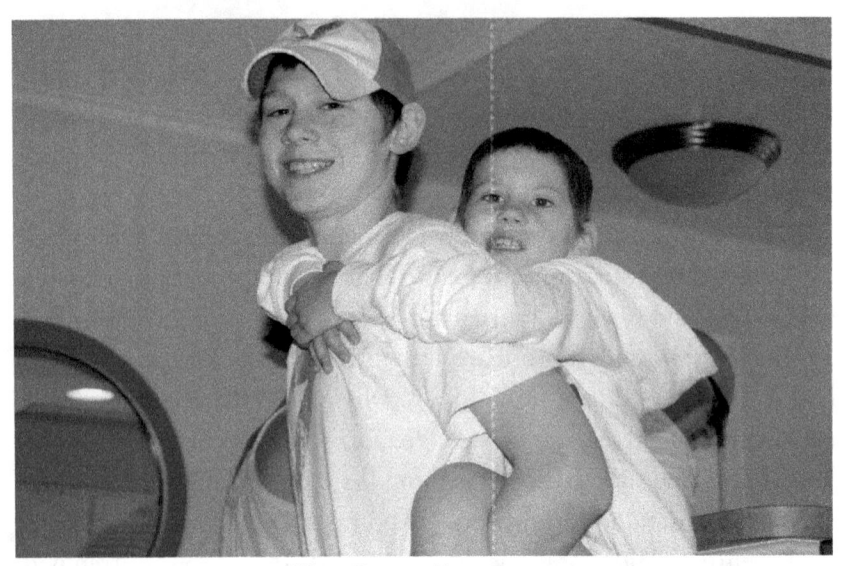

Ethan Brown, Alexa Brown

"Alexa, I love you more than life itself and would give anything to trade you places. Even though you are Heaven and I am still on Earth that doesn't mean I cannot make you a valentine. I know you will see it one way or another. I miss you little sis and can't wait to be with you again in Heaven."

Ethan
On CaringBridge.com

chapter 20

In the following days, there was reaction from the Ohio EPA about Alexa's death.

"It's definitely a tragedy," said OEPA Spokesperson Dina Pierce. Yep. The same Dina Pierce who confirmed the Ohio EPA had dropped the ball early in the study instead of doing the extra testing it promised the community.

"I think we can say (Alexa's death) emphasizes the importance of the work we're doing in trying to find out what's going on," she added, talking about the air and water tests it was conducting. "Old landfill sites…we might want to check into…that might be a possibility," she added. That very statement would prove to be an interesting one. Just remember, she said this in August of 2009.

"What we want to do is look at everything and try to determine what has caused this outbreak in childhood cancers," she said during the taped TV interview. "If it's there, we want to find it and we are going to keep looking and doing everything we can. We are not going to quit until we have exhausted all of our options," she said at that time without knowing what the agency really had in mind for the future of the investigation.

Meanwhile, the federal government had started paying more attention, and the spotlight was about to shine on just how all the agencies involved were handling this cancer cluster. "So, you're planning to be there early in the afternoon on the 12th?" I asked over the phone while sitting at my desk in the newsroom.

"That's the plan," the voice on the other end informed me. "He has another event that morning, but we are planning to be there to talk with the Browns in Clyde," she added.

The "he" was U.S. Senator Sherrod Brown. Sherrod is a taller, younger-than-normal-senator looking man with brown curly hair. His thin frame suggested he was health conscious or perhaps just had good genes. I guessed it was the former. His voice, though, reminded me of a man who had been smoking for 30 years. It's the kind of sound that almost hurts my voice just listening to his tone. The rasp was harsh but his heart was not.

That August day was hot. I remember stepping out of our live van and instantly beads of sweat started to form on my brow. The sun was bright and my sunglasses provided a bit of protection from the elements.

We set up on that familiar front porch. Camera perched on the tri-pod pointing toward the cul-du-sac so we could capture the senator's arrival. Several cars started to approach and then stopped at the Brown's house.

Out of a car steps Senator Brown. His shirtsleeves rolled up to his elbows.

"You Warren?" the senator asked as he approached the front porch of the Browns home. Thankfully, the roof of the porch created some much-needed shade. The senator extended his hand.

"I'm Warren," the big, bald father said, with what I can only imagine was a very firm handshake that alone told the senator that Warren was happy to see him there. And that Warren was serious about this meeting.

"This is my wife, Wendy," said Warren, pointing to his better half.

"Hi, Wendy. I'm Sherrod Brown," he said shaking her hand, too.

"I know who you are," Wendy said with a smile and a turn of the head showing the senator that she, too, was glad to see him make the trip.

There I was with Shawn rolling the entire time, standing on the porch on a hot summer day, sweating through my long sleeve shirt and tie, and trying not to be noticed as we were taping.

Warren had a game plan for the sitting arrangement on the porch. Beforehand, he told us he wanted to put Sherrod in the far-right corner where the porch ends and the bushes begin. Then he was going to flank the senator with Wendy on the left side and Warren on the right.

"I don't want him to think he can get up and sneak away," explained Warren with a crafty smile before the senator arrived. "I want to be able to corner him so he listens to every word we say," he added while arranging the seats. His plan worked to perfection.

"Senator, please have a seat," Warren said, guiding Sherrod to the corner seat and pointing with his hand straightened out.

Warren had a collared shirt, shorts and bare feet. Yes, this man who was a well-respected public leader in the county and who was hosting a U.S. senator on his front porch to talk about serious issues like childhood cancer, did not have socks or shoes on. He was making a point. He was not a simpleton by any stretch of the imagination, but he was a simple kind of man with a down-home message from the roots of small-town America.

"I think I need to share Alexa's story with you," said Warren with his large arms propped on the arm rests of his chair.

Warren and Wendy bounced back and forth describing all that Alexa and the family had endured during the past three years. It wasn't a long story, but it was full of details to let the senator know the severity of her case.

"This past Easter Sunday, all of a sudden Alexa's legs started to hurt her," said Wendy, wearing a thin, comfortable shirt on the heat-filled afternoon. "Within two weeks, she couldn't walk," the mother explained.

Wendy continued with a description about their recent trip to Vermont and the devastating news they got about the return of Alexa's cancer. She talked about the lack of blood services available for home care and how family and friends watched over Alexa just inside the walls that Sherrod's back was facing.

"Pediatrics has always been underfunded," the senator said after patiently listening to every word the concerned parents shared. He sat in the corner with his legs crossed, elbows on the armrests, and his hands together in an upside-down V formation. His fingers touched each other near his face. "NIH (National Institutes of Health) gets 31 billion dollars. NCI (National Cancer Institute) is part of NIH and I don't think Congress will ever say to NIH 'you need to spend it on these diseases.' But they will begin to say—and they should say—you need to spend more in pediatrics," he commented.

Senator Brown talked about how he wanted a special center of excellence at pediatric hospitals around the country. He wanted one or two in Ohio to get things going to get more attention paid to pediatrics. He was working on a bill with the Cincinnati Children's Hospital.

Warren then addressed the recent bill signed into law called the Carolyn Pryce Walker Conquer Childhood Cancer Act. President Barrack Obama penned it on July 29, 2008 after it passed without opposition in the House and Senate. It was supposed to appropriate 30 million dollars a year for five years specifically for childhood cancer research and treatments. At the time that the senator sat on that porch in Clyde, it was August of 2009 and no money had been released.

"NCI should be spending tens and tens and tens of millions on pediatrics," said Senator Brown.

"Well, the act itself is written for 30 million dollars a year for five years so it needs to be at least that and it should be more," Warren chimed in.

"30 million dollars can go a long way in putting a lot of people to work in 200 research centers across the country," Sherrod said

"So, I'm guessing based on what you've said, you're a proponent of this?" asked Warren.

"Yes. I am, yes," said the senator sitting next to the couple and moving his head so both could see his smile.

"Wonderful," said Warren, throwing a similar smile right back at the man who was in a very important position in our nation's capital. "The kids have always had to take a backseat. What I'm hearing you say today is that they're not going to take a backseat anymore?" Warren questioned.

"That's right," said Sherrod. "That's right."

Wendy grabbed a picture of Alexa and showed it to the senator. "Six times she lost her hair," she said as the photo showed the bald little girl's head and that famous crooked smile.

"She had beautiful eyes," the senator smiled while holding the picture in his hands. I could tell as he looked into those eyes of Alexa, he was probably thinking about his own daughters. I could also tell he was taking a moment to absorb what he had just heard from the Browns.

After about an hour-long visit, it was time for Sherrod to return to the road. I pulled him aside for an interview.

"Give me your initial reaction to what the Browns told you here on their porch today," I said holding the microphone and Shawn burning the images onto our digital tape.

"They've been through the worst possible experience that I can imagine," he told me, reflecting on the stories of Alexa. "What I need to do now is go down to Washington and talk to the right people in the appropriations committee and work with the health committee on which I sit and talk to leadership in both parties," explained the senator. "Make sure we can take this step, not the biggest step, but an important beginning step," he told me, talking about getting the funding released for the Carolyn Pryce Walker Conquer Childhood Cancer Act.

"So, what's your message to the families in our area who are dealing with these cancer cases?" I asked.

"I hope the children lead long lives," he said. "You never have enough resources, but you can really, really explore some of the resources and help people like this one (cluster) in Clyde," he answered.

"So, you're going to be committed?" I questioned.

"Of course, I am," the senator said with a convincing tone and a straight look at me. I have seen shifty responses before from politicians who want to just say what the people want to hear without believing it themselves. I did not see that from Senator Brown.

After the interview, the senator said that he really appreciated our dedication to this story. He told me his wife wrote for the Cleveland Plain Dealer and had reported on many health issues in past articles.

The senator, with his staff members in tow, got back into the car and drove away. It was the same direction Alexa's hearse took, but the Browns had a little more confidence in what was to come from this departure.

"He seemed to be paying a lot of attention to us and he asked some critical questions," said Warren during our post front-porch summit interview.

"He seemed genuinely concerned," noted Wendy. "He seemed like he is going to push for more funding…like he really cared," she added.

"I was glad to see him come back to my point about how the government needs to be pointed in a certain direction. You need to tell these folks where to spend the money," said Warren.

"This can't wait a decade to start doing something," Wendy emphasized during our interview.

By the end of our discussion on camera, it all came full circle back to Alexa…as it should.

"Her journey, although it may be over in an earthly fashion, there's a new path that's just opened up," Warren said with a smile that told me he was pleased with today's meeting.

That night on the 11 o'clock show, our anchor Jerry Anderson delivered the news. "It's a day a Clyde family has been waiting for…a chance to tell political leaders to push for more funding for childhood cancer research…"

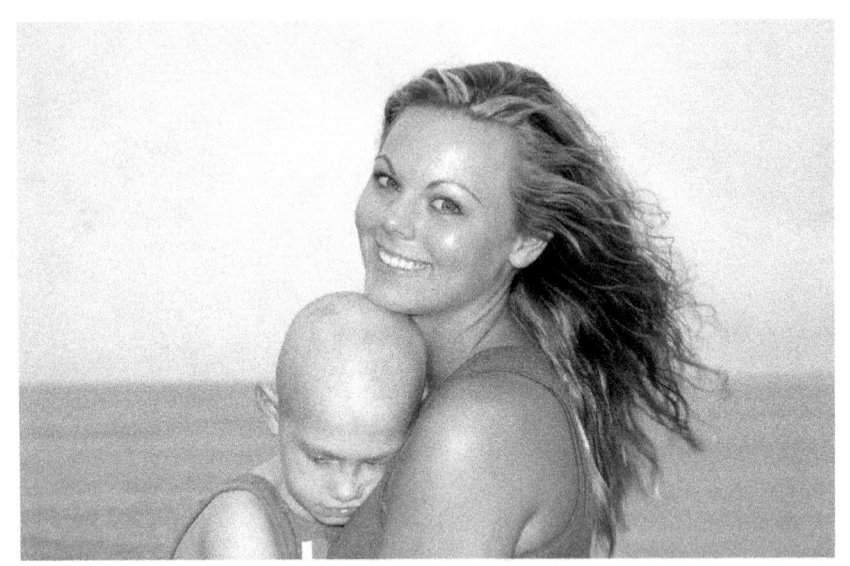

Alexa Brown, Amanda Brown

"Someone recently mentioned to Amanda if she was 'moving on'. This person is one who evidently has never lost a child of a baby sister. For those who have had this experience the fact remains that one never truly moves on. Of course, we (the collective 'we—the Browns') continue to live life, go to work, watch our other kids get married or go to college but they, along with us, will always remain bound to that time when our 'little sis' was still part of our earthly existence."

Warren
On CaringBridge.com

chapter 21

Three days after that meeting with Sherrod Brown, it was time to celebrate Alexa's life. A day to remember the girl so many had supported and who inspired so many. It was time to lay Alexa to rest.

The sun was out and, during our now very familiar drive to Clyde, I noticed my photographer Shawn had dressed up for the occasion. "Look at you with your fancy pants on," I said taking a jab at his normal work attire—jeans and the occasional inappropriate wording on T-shirts and sweatshirts. Today, he had on a nice pair of pants and a button-down shirt. "I do what I can," he fired back with a smirk and a brief chuckle. His laugh always made me laugh. It was contagious and I needed to catch that because I knew this day was not going to be fun.

"How do you want to do this?" asked Shawn talking about the approach we were going to take to this news story. We often would have a "game plan talk" during our drives just to get a sense of what each of us was thinking about the coverage we were about to undertake.

"Well," I said searching for thoughts on how this should be different from all the other funerals I had covered in the past. "I gotta think the church is going to be packed. So, we will need to find a place to set up, stay out of the way, and get everyone fulfilling their roles during the ceremony. It could be a bit difficult," I concluded.

At the same time, I tried to imagine the shots we needed to show our audience the dichotomy of the service. On the one hand, we had all lost an incredible young lady who touched so many lives. Even thinking about her not being alive anymore was hard to deal with. So, that sadness was bound to be a part of the event. On the other hand, the lessons we had all learned through such a powerful, yet weak-bodied girl was something to celebrate. I knew I had to accomplish both goals in one story that would last only two minutes. Never let it be said there are not challenges to television journalism.

As we pulled up in our Jeep Liberty about 45 minutes before the ceremony, there were cars already lined up around the church. It was a warm mid-August day. As we got our camera out of the car, I noticed a constant trickle of people dressed in lightly colored clothing. Some had their ties on, others shirts and sport coats, and dresses that looked more like Easter Sunday attire. Those who really knew Alexa, wore her favorite color purple.

We walked into the church and there was no place to sit. Row after row people sat and fanned themselves with the paper funeral programs trying to beat the late summer heat seeping in from the outside.

"What if we went to the side, sort of in the middle of the right aisle?" asked Shawn who was trying to pinpoint the best location for our camera.

"Let's take a look from the balcony, too, just in case you want to take the camera off the tripod," I added.

As we made our way around the church searching for locations, we were definitely noticed by those sitting in the pews. Some eyes that made contact with ours, followed up with a smile. Others did not. There were times during our overall coverage that I would hear from the families who we focused on in our stories that some citizens of Clyde did not appreciate our reports. They thought we were focusing on the negative aspects of the town that had this horrible mystery.

They didn't understand the motives of the Hiseys or the Browns who consistently stepped forward to keep this topic on the forefront of everyone's mind. They did not realize that these families had many goals when it came to childhood cancer. In fact, Dave Hisey ran the local grocery store in Clyde. He told me the story of a woman who actually stopped him in the store and told him he was more interested in being on TV than taking care of his sick children.

Can you imagine? He told me it took every ounce of self-restraint not to lash out against the woman. I couldn't blame him. He eventually told the old woman that he would give anything in the world to not be in his situation.

These parents were courageous people not only fighting for their kids but others, too. They were fighting to hold people accountable in the agencies responsible for finding the cause and stopping the spread of cancer to other families in the community. Some of the stares in the church that day left me feeling like my motives were not understood either.

After scoping the entire layout of the church, we decided on the far-right aisle just enough behind a pillar. The camera was tucked away and not so obvious. We then went back to the balcony to sit and wait for the service. When we got up there, Warren and Amanda were already there sitting next to the organ. We gave them each a hug.

"The church looks great," I said, trying to break the obvious torture Warren was feeling. He was looking down and picking at his hands. "Lots of people are here. That's great, Warren," I added, searching for that positive eye contact. I did not get it.

"These are great people who've supported us through all of this," he said continuing to play with his large hands. These were the same hands that tried so hard to take care of the little girl who he was about to bury.

He abruptly got up and left the balcony. It was not a negative reaction, but I think he just didn't know what to do. What do you do as you wait for your daughter's funeral? I don't know. Play with your hands maybe and think. So much time left now to think.

"I just remember how I wanted to make sure everything was perfect," said Warren looking back at the day. "I wanted everything to be perfect. Not for me but so that Alexa's memorial service would be something that people never ever forget," he added. More tears slid down his cheek.

"There's a picture that we took before we all went to the church," remembered Wendy about that morning. "We had cousins and all kinds of family there at the house. There we were standing on the porch and it was just surreal. Here we were all smiling and Alexa was not there. Of course, we all knew Alexa was in Heaven, but every time I look at that picture, it's like she should have been there and our family would have been at our home for some other reason.

There would have been an earthly reason to smile, not just us thinking about our little girl who had passed away and who is now standing beside God," she added.

Frank Brown was Alexa's uncle. He was also a minister. He was assigned the difficult task of officiating the service of his young niece. He was a tall, healthy man with a similar build to Warren's. He was dressed in a black robe with a butterfly laden stole.

Just before the service started, the Browns came down the center aisle and filled their assigned pew single file. At this point, we were near our camera and could see the expressions on Warren, Abby, Amanda and Ethan. All looked cried out, but you knew there would be more tears surfacing. Wendy made her way to the piano that was in the right corner of the altar. She wanted to play one last time for her daughter.

Shortly after the family took their seats, there was a calmer-than-normal hush that came over the church. It only lasted a moment, but the silence was so intense it could be felt. The time had come for the beginning of the end.

"There came a girl who was sent from God," Frank Brown started. He smiled and moved his head and eyes around the packed church. "Her name was Alexa," he continued with that same smile. "Help us to also celebrate with her, her release from this world, her coming home to you, Father, the One who gave her to us."

Wendy filled the room with beautiful sounds from that piano. Her musical talents never meant so much. Her previous involvement with the church choir or her past music lessons she had given to kids at their home were all important. However, they were nowhere near as important as playing one last time for her little girl.

As that music streamed through the air, my eyes were drawn to the large screen just off to the left side of the altar. It showed pictures of butterflies—Alexa's favorite creatures. It also showed various rotating images of a healthy Alexa before the cancer and even some dramatic shots of her after the disease took over. The people in the church were singing. I was not. I was mesmerized with the frames of Alexa's life including one particular black and white photo. It showed a bald Alexa facing her sister Amanda. Their beautiful faces filled the screen.

Their heads leaned close together in the middle of the frame. Smiles adorned their faces as they looked into each other's eyes.

As the song ended, there was a brief pause. Abby then approached the podium. She had a poem to read.

"She enters God's world a new and vibrant child. No more pain. No more tears and no more fears," the oldest sister read aloud. A large sigh exited her worn body…weathered from the tears that were once again making an appearance on her lovely face. "God accepts her and keeps her safe. When the sun sets and you're ready to rest, she'll be near to say 'Good night, sleep tight, don't let the bed bugs bite.' I'm here beside you in your dreams, in your memories, in your thoughts and in your heart," Abby continued through the obvious emotion of the moment. She looked up at the crowd and said, "Thank you for loving my sister."

Wendy then started playing Amazing Grace. The congregation joined in the song that was filled with so much more meaning when applied to Alexa. "I once was lost, but now am found. Was blind but now I see." At one point she was seeing double when the first signs of this terrible disease reared its ugly head, but now all of that was behind her. Alexa had lost her body to cancer but her spirit found its way to God.

Soon after Amazing Grace, it was time for Ethan to take the altar for a reading. Warren had told me before the ceremony that he did not know if Ethan could make it through his portion of the service. We were about to find out.

As the tall teenager with a young face but a strong, athletic build stepped to the podium, even his muscular physique could not hold up under the emotion of his sister's passing. "The Lord is my shepherd, I shall not want," he managed to get out while looking down and speaking with a weakened voice. There was a long pause. The ever-familiar tears were too strong for this tough child to hold back. He shook his head, turned to his uncle, and threw his arms around his Uncle Frank for a hug that said, "I just can't do this." Frank just smiled and completed the reading: Psalm 23.

"The Lord is my shepherd. I shall not want. He maketh me to lie down in green pastures: He leadeth me beside the still waters.

He restoreth my soul: He leadeth me in the paths of the righteousness for His name's sake. Yet, though I walk through the valley of the shadow of death, I will fear no evil: for Thou art with me; the rod and the staff comfort me. Thou preparest a table before me in the presence of mine enemies; Thou anointest my head with oil; my cup runneth over. Surely goodness and mercy shall follow me all the days of my life: and I will dwell in the house of the Lord forever," Frank recited. I cannot tell you how many times I have heard that very verse, but I can tell you how closely I listened this time to each word and how they related to Alexa's Journey.

Warren made his way to the front of the church. He gave his brother a huge hug and read a different passage. "I will rejoice in Jerusalem and delight in my people and the sound of weeping and crying will be heard in it no more," the father of Alexa said. At the end of the reading, he added his own words. "Alexa has fought the good fight. Alexa has finished her race and she did remain faithful," he told the crowd. Many heard the words and nodded in agreement.

Amanda was next in the ceremony. She called everyone's attention to the video screen that had been showing photos. It was time for a video. The tape showed Alexa at the tender age of four. She was sitting at a table outside right next to her cousin Emily. They were playing a game of tag while sitting there.

"Tag. You're it," said Alexa.

"Tag. YOU'RE it," shouted Emily.

The two then just started touching each other over and over again. "Tag, tag, tag, tag, tag," they said in unison. The entire audience erupted in laughter and relished in the beauty that emanated from the children. The video ended and smiles filled the room.

"I remember holding Alexa in the hospital," recalled Amanda. "Her falling asleep in my arms and thinking I'm so glad this little baby is now my little sister. She was beautiful inside and out and she was the most important person of my life," continued the big sis. She went on to talk about a special memory…a particular hug. "It was one of those bear hugs where she just wouldn't let go. It was one of those hugs where you didn't want to let go. As her arms were still wrapped tightly around my neck, she whispered in my ear, 'I love you so much.' This is who Alexa was. She had a heart that could burst with love at any moment. She was gentle and strong and she loved me with her whole heart as I loved her with my whole heart," Amanda shared.

She also talked about a recent entry in the CaringBridge journal. "She has touched thousands of people and she has battled this cancer with such grace," Amanda read with her eyes now filled with tears. "I want to keep her forever. I want to kiss her and hug her and rest my head on her lap when I'm not feeling well." She ended with these words: "I love you, family and friends, but most of all I love you, Alexa."

Alexa did touch thousands of people through the CaringBridge journal entries (which you will find some journal entries here throughout the book) and through the news coverage about her battle. Her Uncle Frank talked about that next.

"In fighting the fight herself, she didn't want others to be pulled down or hurt in any way," the minister said with a comforting smile. "That's fighting the good fight. She set a good example for you and for me to fight the good fight, to keep fighting in this world that caused this suffering and I trust you are committed to that fight," he said looking out at those seated before him.

The minister read from one of the many letters Alexa got from strangers. This one was from a single mother. "I started reading your journal and it inspired me to stop feeling sorry for myself and become the best mother and person that I could be." A girl not even in her teens inspired people three, four, five times her age to be strong. Alexa, herself was not physically strong, but somehow she realized she had to be emotionally fit to keep others in the right frame of mind.

That photo of her head next to Amanda's became such a symbol at that moment for me. The wear and tear took out her locks of hair, but what was inside was an unscathed spirit that remained strong despite the tangible troubles. As she was pictured leaning into Amanda's eyes, she showed she did lean on her family, but she also transferred her strength for them to carry on this war against childhood cancer.

"She leaves us the witness. She leaves us the challenge," said Frank. "Will you fight the good fight?" he asked with raised eyebrows.

"It's a life that we will remember and continue to celebrate," added the minister. "The life of Alexa Katherine Brown."

As the service ended, the crowd gathered outside of the church in a large grassy area. White and purple balloons were handed out and then released at the same time. The floating bubbles became silhouettes as they crossed right in front of the bright sun. The rays danced around the ovals as they went further and further into the immaculate, blue sky. All eyes were raised recognizing the symbolism and knowing Alexa was in a better place. It was a perfect ending to a memorable ceremony, though, every single person wished a healthy Alexa would have stayed with us much longer.

"It really was a perfect memorial service, but it's not anything that any parent should have to go through ever," said Warren in retrospect. "We're not the only ones who have done this. It happens every day."

"These are things that should be preventable. In this country we have the brightest minds, wonderful scientists, great doctors, tremendous researchers, but if you don't give them the tools to do their jobs then you're not going to find an answer to this every day problem," he added.

The next night after our funeral piece aired, we put together another report. It was a revelation Wendy had shared with us that I just happened to find while logging our tapes from the days leading up to the funeral. When I found it, I knew it would be a nice follow-up to some of the messages given at the funeral.

"Welcome to News 11, I'm Jonathan Walsh," I said looking into the studio camera. I was anchoring the news that Sunday night. "A day after the community of Clyde said goodbye to Alexa Brown, the family says perhaps questions ARE being answered about her journey. News 11 has been following Alexa's journey even giving the family a camera when they went to Vermont looking to get Alexa into a drug trial. That trip to the Vermont Children's Hospital revealed another brain tumor and the family came right back home. Well, now Alexa's mother says there WAS a reason for that trip," I told the audience while they watched video of Alexa's battle with cancer.

Wendy's soundbite then came up. "I've been trying to figure out the point of why we went to Vermont and all the trouble that came from that trip," Wendy said explaining the constant thoughts that went through her mind. "But that trip started the video blog with Channel 11. That's what was good. Through Channel 11, the bigger picture is now being seen," Wendy said with her arms raised and spread apart symbolizing the bigger picture.

After the soundbite, I continued reading on camera. "Because of those blogs, the family says they have received letters and emails from people around the country who've followed Alexa's story and have been inspired by her strength. Plus, they helped political leaders see the need for more funding," I said finishing the story.

The bigger question was just how much would the politicians be motivated by the courageous journey of a little girl from a tiny town named Clyde in Ohio? It was clear to the Brown family. They had to keep this in the spotlight.

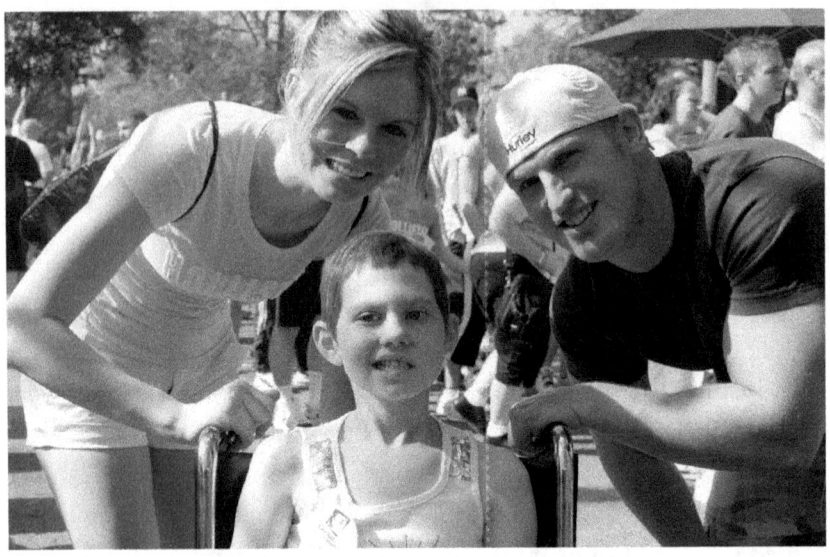

Abby Brown, Alexa Brown, Greg Reynolds

"Alexa's birthday—belief and acceptance of her physical absence is barely overcome by knowing she is whole and perfect. Still, she would have all of us continue on and become the best we can become. This we must do in honor of her legacy."

Warren
On CaringBridge.com

chapter 22

In the days following Alexa's final celebration, it looked like people were moved into action. We caught word of Senator Sherrod Brown's further commitment to finding funds for pediatric cancer research. We did a story about Warren asking everyone who was touched by Alexa's journey to write to his or her senators.

By the early days of September, we were reminding people that it was National Childhood Cancer Awareness Month. I passed out gold ribbons for the anchors to wear during their shows. "Tonight, we're wearing these ribbons in honor of Alexa Brown who lost her battle with cancer last month," they announced to our viewers. The gold ribbon is recognized as a symbol of childhood cancer awareness. I wore one every day.

At one point, I heard about the ribbon-making parties that were popping up at the home of the Browns. Family and friends spent hours on end preparing ribbons and spreading the word at local events. I had to do a story.

"A lot of love goes into these things," said Amanda who was sitting at the dining room table with five other young people. They had glue guns, spools of gold ribbons, numerous scissors, and small gold safety pins. There were also small square pieces of paper with words on them describing the importance of the gold ribbons. The kids were attaching the ribbons to the papers.

"We've made a pretty good amount so far," Amanda said with drips of dried glue all over her fingers and tiny red marks where the hot glue gun had accidentally made contact with her skin. All of the kids had those red marks.

My report showed just some of the six thousand ribbons the volunteers made and then handed out at various locations in Clyde including a recent Clyde-Bellevue football game. They were not selling the ribbons but rather taking what people could give in return; money, hugs, whatever. It didn't matter. They just wanted to keep the cancer cause on people's minds.

"I love my sister very much and I need to do what I can to help other kids. Seeing Alexa die was too much," Amanda told us all while continuing the glue dots, ribbon cutting, and pin-piercing assembly line at the table.

As the volunteers went on spreading the message, the Browns got word that Senator Sherrod Brown planned a speech on the senate floor that would encourage other senators to act on funding for pediatric cancer research. It was good news and that seemed to pull additional students into the political aspect of this fight.

At one point when I had a day off, one of our reporters Justin Michaels did a story about how kids at Clyde schools were writing letters to Washington, D.C.

"It's been part of our lives for the past few years and I want to see it change," said one teen. They called it the "Charge for Change" that involved students from elementary to high school penning their thoughts that would eventually be faxed to congressional leaders. They asked for more funding.

Teachers and administrators were impressed. "I think this gave our students a chance to voice their opinion when they usually wouldn't have that opportunity," said one adult. "People didn't just take this as an assignment. People really put their hearts into the letters," commented another.

Warren was excited that Alexa's journey played a role in the students' increased awareness and action. "800 students wrote letters. That brought me to tears when I started thinking about the efforts behind what these young people have done," Warren told us. "Alexa was a catalyst. I mean, she got this started but this is for all the children around here who have suffered through this," he added.

It turned out that 2000 letters flooded fax machines in Washington.

The constant feeding forced district offices to turn their machines off. Message heard.

Students well beyond the Clyde area dove into the funding push, too. Fifth grader Jase Whitner from Perrysburg, Ohio didn't even know Alexa but he saw all the news coverage. He decided he could do something.

"Some kids just have to go through that and it's just sad," the 10-year-old told us. He accepted donations on Alexa's behalf at a booth he set up right in the middle of a book fair and "Family Fun Night" at Toth Elementary School. One of those kids who went through the same fight was seven-year-old Maddie Trudel. She passed away in 2006.

Maddie was not a part of the cancer cluster, but her aunt Maggie Laube from Perrysburg helped take care of the little girl during that 18-month fight against cancer. "She was a very dynamic young lady like Alexa and she had a really good heart and touched a lot of people," said Maggie. She was at the school and made a donation to Jase's cause.

Another concerned parent, Jon Hawker, got a gold ribbon from Jase, too. "There's a lot of good causes out there," Hawker said while handing the ribbon to his young daughter. "Everyone's got to fight their fight and looks like he's picked a good one," he added.

All around Jase, there were booths full of children getting their faces painted, playing games, and getting snacks. All of that was so much more fun than setting up a table focused on cancer, but none of the other activities fazed him. He thought about the Browns and so did Jase's principal. "Your heart goes out to them and you want to do everything you can to help," Principal Beth Christoff told me while standing in front of the young man's display.

Jase had a message for the Browns. "I hope you guys feel better," the young man told us. He was a kid right around Alexa's age when she passed away. Children can understand and, clearly, Jase got it.

Someone else who got it? Sherrod Brown. He worked behind the scenes ever since that sit-down meeting on Warren and Wendy's front porch. By the end of September, he was informing his fellow senators about Alexa's journey. On September 30, 2009 he took to the microphone on the senate floor and told everyone about the special girl from northwest Ohio and her family.

"Alexa Brown was an active, happy little girl," described the raspy-voiced senator in front of his colleagues. He talked about how cancer stole the little girl's body from her and eventually ended her life. "As you can imagine, it was an emotional time for them and for their friends, and for their neighbors, and for their friends at church and their friends throughout Clyde. Even in their state of mourning, Alexa's mom and dad stressed the importance of making sure other families don't have to go through this same ordeal," he explained. He also told the powerful politicians that cancer is the number one cause of non-accidental death among children. Number one. He encouraged Congress to support more funding for childhood cancer research while reminding members that Alexa's scenario was "not an isolated case".

Right after that speech, more reports surfaced about additional steps people in our nation's capital were taking. Senators Sherrod Brown and George Voinovich co-signed a first-of-its-kind letter urging the Senate Appropriations Committee to approve millions of dollars specifically for pediatric cancer research. The momentum was on track. At least it appeared that way.

It was as if someone turned the faucet on and flooded awareness of the importance of childhood cancer research. Just like water that combines a bunch of little drops to make a full stream, there were a lot of little pieces of this cancer puzzle starting to fit together. Parents and kids. Students and teachers. Local voters and national politicians. The dam to this water flow, though, came from the state level.

"New at 11…after calls from news 11 and pushing from parents, it appears there will be more information released about the childhood cancer cluster," said anchor Jerry Anderson one October night. "Some of the families involved have been asking for a detailed map locating where the cancer victims live. The Ohio Department of Health originally said it could not release that information because of privacy issues. News 11 recently spoke to the man helping to spearhead the study asking if families could sign a waiver if they wanted their info released. Warren Brown tells News 11 that the health department's chief of staff told him forms would be coming to all families who can either opt in or opt out of the map. Some of the families say the map is crucial for their own studies into what has caused 37 children to get cancer in that area," Jerry said finishing the brief update for our viewers.

This new "change of heart" by the department of health meant a new meeting was going to happen once again at the Sandusky County Health Department in Fremont. I sat, again in that same parking lot I had become all too familiar with as the private meetings were going on inside. At least I knew this time, I would be able to ask some serious questions to Robert Indian and Dina Pierce. I did not think I could be surprised again by what was happening with the study. I was wrong. I hate being wrong.

In between the time of the announcement of the meeting and the actual get together, I got a call from Steve Keller. He was the grandfather of Kole Keller, a little boy was a part of the study and who passed away from cancer.

"Jonathan, I want to talk to you about what's going on," said the low-toned, harsh-whispered voice on the other end of the line. "There's too much red tape. There's too much that people aren't doing to find the problem here," Steve said very seriously. "You want to come over to the house?" he asked.

This was the same man who had not said a word to me for the past couple of years other than one, quick phone conversation. It was an important conversation; one that told me he was contacting Erin Brockovich's law firm for help. Now, as he asked me to come over to his house, I remembered that I asked him in that previous short phone call if I would be able to talk to him later when he was ready. He told me then that he would think about it. Apparently, he thought about it.

"Absolutely, Steve," I told the grandfather. "I would love to sit down with you and you can tell me whatever you want about the research you've done and how much Kole meant to you," I added.

"Something needs to be done," he said sternly.

We set up a time to talk at his home in Oak Harbor, Ohio.

I hung up the phone and walked to the office of my news director. "Andi, I have an idea," I told her as she was sitting at her desk.

I informed her about the new interview with Steve and the upcoming meeting with the families. I thought I could combine the two for an expanded story during our November ratings period. That way we could promote the piece and draw more attention to these new elements.

"Let's do it," Andi said to me.

When the video rolled for the news that night, soft music started as it faded up from black to a picture of Kole. He was a little boy with short hair, wearing a nice shirt and a smile that would light up any room. His eyes made you look right into them. His light skin against his dark hair gave such a contrast to his overall appearance that you could not help but notice his handsome face. There was a different contrast as well, that such a beautiful child would have such an ugly fate.

"Kole Keller was just four years old when he was diagnosed with a brain tumor," my voice began on the report. "Kole's grandfather, Steve Keller, is opening up for the first time in-depth about his grandson losing his fight to cancer just two days after Kole turned six," I told the audience as they watched Steve sitting on his small couch.

Steve was in his late 50's or early 60's with a bald head that was dotted with sunspots. I could tell he spent a lot of time outdoors. He was shorter than my 5'11" frame, but he was in much better shape than I was. His lean body was toned and just beyond his short-sleeved shirt, the definition of his muscles could clearly be seen. He was physically strong and healthy. His grandson was not.

"That's one of the reasons…excuse me," Steve said, as this older, pillar of strength started to show cracks in his emotional walls. Tears welled up as he thought back on the grandson he loved so much. "I wanted to research this because two days before he passed, he had a birthday cake with Spiderman, Superman and I think Batman… superheroes," Steve remembered. He couldn't complete the thought. His stare was blank but very much full of meaning.

"Steve says Kole was his own superhero for other children battling cancer," my voice continued on tape. "There was a time when doctors at St. Jude's Hospital in Tennessee treated Kole. Steve recalled one specific day at a Memphis Church," I continued as photos of Kole passed on screen. Kole without hair. Kole in hospital gowns. Kole in the throes of that dreadful battle called cancer.

"The pastor asked, 'What do you need?' Kole answered, 'I want you to pray for all the kids at St. Jude's Hospital,'" recounted the little boy's grandfather who understandably gave no fight against the emotion of his memories. More tears made their way down Steve's strong face. "He was a loving kid. He didn't just care about himself. He cared about others," Steve told us as he took his small, black-rimmed glasses off with one hand and wiped his now red cheeks with the other.

I then showed a picture of Kole sitting in a hospital bed looking directly at the camera. "This is Kole holding his baby brother, Judah," I explained. "Judah was born just a week before Kole passed away. It was the first time Kole had smiled in about a month," my voice narrated. Those last few days for Kole were nothing to smile about, but at least he got the chance to see his brother and hold him like a "normal" sibling.

"We need to do this, figure this out to help future kids," said Steve. "We need to find out what's going on," he uttered with an even more serious tone.

The next video showed an old Rand McNally map of Sandusky County. It was a used, tattered, creased lined map that I started poking with pushpins marking the cases of childhood cancer.

"For the past few months, family members of the kids involved with this cancer study have been asking the Ohio Department of Health for the department's completed, detailed map showing where the cancer victims have lived," I told our viewers. "The families tell News 11 the map could help them research where water sources are in relation to the victims, where industrial sites are and so forth. The Ohio Department of Health said it couldn't release that information because of patient privacy issues. So, both the families and News 11 asked if a waiver form could be signed by those who wanted their information released. The state said it would look into it," I revealed in the story.

The next shot showed Steve on the couch listening to my question off-camera. "Would you sign a waiver saying, 'Hey, I don't care if people know where I live?'" I said throwing the hypothetical situation out there. "Oh, sure," Steve told me without hesitation.

The next soundbite was from Warren Brown. "Everybody knows where we live. Have we had any issues? No. Has anybody bothered us? No," he said in the taped interview.

Dave Hisey then appeared on the screen. "It just seems like they make it too hard. It's a lot of work to find out information that we should already have," Dave told me in a frustrated tone.

I then showed pictures of the families walking through the chilly fall night at the Sandusky County Health Department. They were filling in for that get-together with the state agencies. "Fast forward about five weeks (from that interview with the families we did with Steve, Warren, and Dave) and this closed-door meeting at the Sandusky County Health Department where the Ohio Department of Health and the Ohio EPA met with the families. After two hours…" I said trailing my voice and leading into the next taped interview.

"One of the decisions we made tonight is that we can produce a map that doesn't require people to sign a waiver," said Robert Indian in that accustomed dark parking lot.

"News 11 asked if the map had already been completed why wasn't it released more quickly," my voice told the audience.

"So far it's been limited to the original 18 folks," answered Robert. "We have not included those folks in Fremont yet. We haven't talked to them. We don't know how long they've been there. The folks in Ottawa County haven't been contacted yet. So, there's a lot of groundwork to lay," Robert explained as I froze the interview on the screen and zoomed into his face. My voice came right back up. "Did you hear that?" I asked the people watching the report. "The Ohio Department of Health hasn't even contacted the 20 other families yet," I said in a surprised-yet-frustrated-toned delivery.

"Let's take you back to this video, May 29th of this year," I said while showing file video of Robert Indian standing and explaining a chart that had a huge circle on a map of eastern Sandusky County. He was standing in front of a group of people in a conference room. "Robert Indian held a meeting describing a bigger circle, a larger area that he and the department were—at the time—including in this study. Five and a half months later, while we were standing in this parking lot, again, the department of health hasn't contacted those additional families," I told the viewers in a way that highlighted my amazement and my "here-we-go-again" tone.

The next portion of video featured Robert's face while I asked another question. "What could be more important than children dying of cancer?" I directed to him.

"I can't think of anything more important," he responded.

"Some of the family members tell us it's not the first time a government agency has let them down," my words continued in my special report, that was now showing the infamous town meeting where Chris Korleski was on the stage at Clyde High School, making his announcement about the new focus on the cluster.

"They say this lack of effort is similar to last year when News 11 exposed the Ohio EPA for going seven months without performing extra testing as promised," I said during the story. "Shortly after our report aired last fall, the Ohio EPA director announced the childhood cancer cluster was its number one priority. Now, during this month's meeting, families received this report," I said showing a wire-spiraled set of papers. "It details what the agencies have done. They've looked at industries and dumpsites and collected water, sediment and air samples," I continued, but none of it really hit home with the families.

"It doesn't give me much hope of them ever finding what caused the cancer," said Trina Donnersbach, who lost her daughter Shilah. "I kind of feel like it's well, let's go through the motions and do what we can do. But really there's not going to be any answers," she added with a noted deflation to her words.

"It's a very slow process," said Dave Hisey. "They're giving us numbers saying this is okay and this seems okay and we can't seem to find anything here. The only things I do know is that we've lost Shilah, Kole, and we've lost Alexa. Now Tanner, my son, is going for a spinal tap tomorrow," Dave described right after the meeting.

"And hope had not looked good at the federal level either," I continued in my story. "News 11 poured over thousands of house bills and resolutions from this year. In those documents, representatives spent much more time and your tax dollars deciding who should be on the next stamp, recognizing golfers, County Music Month, even declaring a resolution for something called 'Complaint-Free Wednesday', than they did recognizing children with cancer," I reported. I showed the viewers numerous specific documents of how our politicians were wasting their time on our dime and at the expense of things that really matter.

"It's crazy," said Steve in reaction to me telling him the list of items elected "leaders" were spending time on. "It doesn't make sense," he said shaking his head in disbelief.

My report rolled on. "Steve tells us the cancer cluster has been so baffling that he met Erin Brockovich in 2006 and told her his story," my voice said as we showed pictures of the rags-to-results attorney with a worldwide reputation for fighting cancer cases just like the one we had in northwest Ohio.

"She's put us in touch with some people," Steve commented. "We've talked. It's a slow process there, too, but Erin's been very helpful."

When Steve told me that, I immediately started thinking about what those meetings were like. He was sitting down, talking to lawyers and, in this case, a high-profile attorney. Describing how your grandson suffered and how more children in your own backyard are suffering and dying. That was happening when all Steve really should have been doing was hitting the water across the street from his home and fishing on his boat with Kole who should still be here on this earth.

"On the wall of Steve's home hangs a saying…'When someone you love becomes a memory, the memory becomes a treasure," I said on tape showing the framed quote. Kole's picture was right beside it. "Steve is fighting for his treasure…Kole…so that his grandson's passing is not in vain," my words finished.

"I think he would be proud of us looking into it," speculated Steve about his grandson, who he believes is sitting in Heaven. "I don't think he'd come back now even if he could because I think he's that happy. But I think he wants to help other kids," the strong grandfather concluded with a sniffle and a few more tears.

I then came back out on camera to end the story with a final thought and a new announcement that would take this fight in a completely new direction.

"The families involved with this study want to help other children as well," I said looking into the large studio camera. "Warren and Wendy Brown from Clyde, who lost their daughter Alexa to cancer in August, are in Washington, D.C. right now. They will be canvassing the Hill encouraging representatives and senators to provide more focus and federal funding for childhood cancer research. I will be there with them and tell you what happens."

Yup. The Browns were going to our nation's capital and I was going to be there, too, every step of the way.

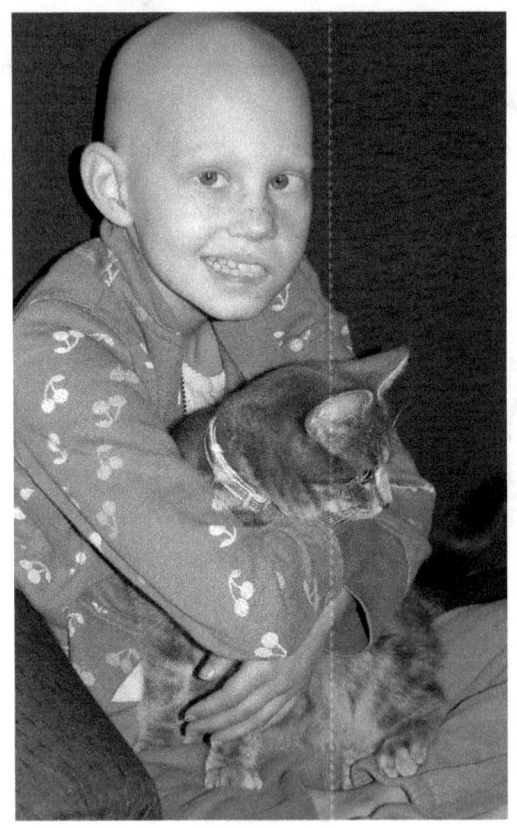

Alexa Brown

"The approximate cost of a Tomahawk cruise missile is $560K. Do you think we could buy 56 less missile, still be secure, and fund the Caroline Pryce Walker Act of 2008? One mile of road renovation costs approximately $750K-1M. Do you think we could pave 30-60 less miles of road this year and fund the Act? Rhetorical questions but ones that bear thought and answering."

Warren
On CaringBridge.com

chapter 23

I had known for a while the Browns wanted to make the trip to D.C. So, in the weeks prior to their visit, I made calls and wrote emails to all the members of Congress who would be important people to meet.

The Browns had a list of elected leaders they wanted to visit and I came up with my own list as well. I spent hours upon hours trying to set up appointments and letting the staff of the politicians know our cameras would be rolling.

"Senator Harkin's office. How can I help you?"

"Senator Durbin's office. How can I direct your call?"

"Senator Spector's office. What can I do for you today?"

My approach was always the same. "My name is Jonathan Walsh and I have an important story to tell you that I know the senator can help out," I would say.

The typical response: "Who are you?"

"I work for the CBS affiliate in Toledo, Ohio. We have a childhood cancer cluster in our area where kids are dying. We've been following it for years and now we're coming to Washington to talk to senators and members of the House who can help these children and their families," I said, not allowing them to interrupt.

The people answering the phones would typically transfer me to the politician's media relations department. Sometimes I got the person who sounded sympathetic. "Oh, that sounds heartbreaking," some told me as I got into Alexa's journey and the cluster itself. "So, what are you wanting from the senator?" others asked matter-of-factly. Then others told me, "The senator doesn't meet with anyone outside of his district."

It's a dirty detail that you may not have known. There are major issues facing all of us and these people make decisions for the entire country, not just their neck of the woods. There are politicians who could care less about meeting with people like the Browns because the Browns will not help get them elected again. I can understand if the topic of my story was funding some project in Toledo, Ohio or more attention was needed for the development of our county. Those are very specific beneficial projects that affect our area only. However, when there are about 4,000 children dying of cancer each year and 12,000 new cases being diagnosed, that breaks down to 80 children per state passing away and one new case every 44 minutes nationwide. So, every one-hour TV episode you watch, another child and then some have been given the life-altering diagnosis. Their families' lives change forever, too, but so many of the politicians are too concerned with elections that they do not recognize the importance of saving these families.

So, I guess it should not have surprised me when not one actual senator from another state or one member of the House met personally with the Browns. Not one. Some took the time to let staffers meet with Warren and Wendy. Those staffers would range from high-level personnel to kids just out of college that had a look of "What the hell am I listening to?"

Call after call letting the offices know the Browns were coming with a camera crew in tow, did not result in a single one-on-one meeting with politicians outside of Ohio, but at least they were getting the chance to meet with people on staff and getting to tell their story.

The plan was for my photographer Shawn Dunagan and me to drive to D.C. and meet up with the Browns. They got there about a day before us. Our drive was 8 hours long. Shawn liked to drive. I'm OK with not being behind the wheel, so the arrangement worked out well.

After checking into our hotel, we called the Browns and met up with them for dinner at the hotel's restaurant. As we sat in the dining room, I talked to Warren and Wendy about the research I did about money these politicians have spent on things other than cancer. I was listing all the projects and we were shaking our heads talking about the waste. As our conversation was in mid-stride, up walked a young man in a suit.

"Hi. I couldn't help but overhear your discussion about the waste here in D.C.," he told us.

"Yeah, it's kind of crazy," Warren told him.

"You guys with some kind of media?" he asked.

We then talked about our background and the story we would be covering in the next couple of days.

"My dad was the editor for a newspaper in Indiana pretty much all his life. So, I love hearing about journalists going after good stories," he revealed.

"That's cool. Thanks, man" I said. "What are you doing down here?" I asked.

"I'm working with a lobbying group trying to get some focus on a new medicine that needs FDA approval," he explained.

I thought to myself that this was the type of guy who we were competing with for the attention of reps controlling the purse strings. "Good luck with your meetings," I told him.

"Yeah, same to you guys, too," he said as his eyes panned to the Browns. "I'm sorry about your daughter. You're doing the right thing," he said as he walked away.

We all hit our rooms. We all said good night knowing that we were starting early the next day and it was already midnight.

"Beep. Beep. Beep," the alarm screamed, or at least it felt like that, as the red illuminated 5:00am cast a red hue in the darkened room. Oh, boy. I did not get enough sleep and I started to come down with a cold. Perfect timing.

I got down to the lobby where Wendy, Warren, Shawn and I were going to meet to catch the shuttle to the Capitol Building. Shawn had his big camera ready and I took the heavy tripod in my hands. Warren and Wendy piled into the long van.

"Where are you guys from?" asked the driver, noticing our TV equipment.

"We're from Toledo," Warren told the man.

"We're from a television station covering these guys and their efforts to get more funding for kids with cancer," I explained.

"Oh, that's a good thing," the driver said with a more noticeable accent now.

Shawn sat next to Warren and I was in the row just in front of him. The camera angle was awkward but it showed the van and the seating to help set the stage that the wheels were in motion. It was the day the Browns had been looking forward to for quite some time.

"How are you feeling right now, Warren?" I asked as Shawn focused on a father about to bring his daughter's case to Capitol Hill.

"I feel very good. I feel hopeful," he said looking straight ahead through the front windshield so as not to miss a thing. I could tell he was excited and nervous all at the same time.

"We're hoping we can convince them to do the right thing," he said continuing to look forward and not at me. "The goal is to get a commitment from the legislators that they will fund the Caroline Pryce Walker Act at the level it was intended to be funded and not pass over it this year as they did last year," he said more for the camera, the two other passengers, and the driver because we knew why we were there. It was nice to hear, though. We were all on the same page in a powerful town.

The Browns got out of the van. "Good luck," shouted the driver with a smile. The first steps were happening…literally.

Shawn was rolling. It was a sunny morning full of the hope Warren described on the ride over. Warren's determined walk got ahead of Wendy who was looking at papers trying to figure out which way to go. Warren was just walking. In the background of his stride was the rotunda of the Capitol. The determination was distinctly written on his face. He said nothing. His thoughts were on the mission and on Alexa.

The first stop was Senator Richard Shelby's office. The politician from Alabama was on the Senate Appropriations Committee. It is the very arm that controls the release of discretionary spending to projects. Some call those projects "pork" but, in the case of kids like Alexa, that money could mean the difference between life and death. The Appropriations Committee is commonly known across Washington as one of the top, most influential, powerful committees in Congress. The members of the Senate and House on their respective committees are the Browns' targets on this trip.

As a member of the media, it was interesting to hear the rules of the U.S. Capitol grounds. In a country that touts its enormously open "freedom of the press principles", that was not the case when dealing with the very people we elect. According to the media relations staff at the Capitol Building, we could not set up a tripod. We could not go into a politician's office with the cameras rolling or we would be tossed out. Of the appointments we did have, every single one of the staff members who were from a different state other than Ohio would not allow our cameras in to tape the meeting. In fact, we had to sit outside of the front door if we had a camera in our possession.

I kept thinking what are they afraid of? Are they fearful that the actual people who are supposed to be helping those who do not have a voice will be seen as ignoring funding for sick children? What about all those other projects that do receive funding? Are they worried about those questions? I was not sure, but it really pissed me off that I would not be able to ask.

As we waited for the Browns to come out of their meeting with Shelby's Health and Human Services aide, Shawn and I just looked around. Big, thick, brown doors dotted the long hallways. People dressed to the nines strode the walkways talking to each other, some pointing to papers, others dragging rolling luggage with what I can only assume are important papers or presentations inside. How many "Brown" families were there that day? How many lobbyists were taking their own steps that day? Every day? We were only there a couple of days. How can we compete with that?

The Browns emerged from a different door than the front of Senator Shelby's office where we were waiting. As we made our way to them, I could see a look of "what just happened" on their faces. Shawn's camera started rolling.

"How did it go in there?" I asked.

"She told us that we truly don't have any idea how deep our message has reached thus far," Warren started, looking amazed.

"She said people have been listening," said Wendy picking up where Warren had trailed off. "She said they know who we are," she continued.

I guess I was not surprised to hear those words. I knew Senator Sherrod Brown had brought up Alexa's name on the floor. Plus, others had been contacted by me, by the Browns, and by different reps from government and non-profit agencies, but at the same time, you never really knew if people were listening.

"How does that make you feel?" I asked during the interview.

"On behalf of Alexa, I couldn't feel any better," said Warren. "It's the message that we're preaching on behalf of the 40,000 other families in this country who are suffering with childhood cancer and the 2,500 families that will have or have suffered the loss of a child as a result of cancer. That's why we're doing this, Jonathan," he continued with a tear or two starting to well up. "We're not doing it for us. It's not about Wendy. It's not about Warren. It's about kids with cancer that haven't had a voice forever," he added looking straight into the camera.

"They are getting the message and they believe what we're doing is the right thing to do," said Wendy.

It was the first meeting of the trip. I thought if this kind of reception continues, then we were about to be a part of something very powerful.

"So, you are walking away with a pretty hopeful feeling?" I asked.

"Yes, I am walking away with a very hopeful feeling," said Wendy.

There's a funny feeling about hope, though. There are no guarantees with hope. You can keep it, but you never know what you're going to really accomplish with it.

The Browns had about an hour before their next meeting so they used the time to drop off important information about Alexa and the Caroline Pryce Walker Conquer Childhood Cancer Act. They carried letters, the gold childhood cancer awareness ribbons, and a DVD I put together of the reports we had done covering the courageous girl's fight.

No appointments had been made but that did not stop them from visiting the offices of Senator Judd Gregg from New Hampshire, Senator Kay Bailey Hutchison from Texas, or Senator Herbert Kohl from Wisconsin. Hallway after hallway, door after door, secretary after secretary, the message stayed the same.

"My name's Warren Brown and this is my wife Wendy," we caught on tape. We put a wireless mic on Warren's sport coat and let the camera roll even if we could not fully see what was going on inside that office of Senator Mary Landrieu from Louisiana. "Over the last couple of weeks, I've been emailing and/or faxing to the senator's scheduler," Warren continued in a polite but pointed fashion. Landrieu was one of many who declined even a staffer to meet with the Browns about kids dying from cancer. "We're canvassing the Hill today on behalf of childhood cancer issues. I know that the senator is on the Appropriations Committee," Warren told the women. He and Wendy stood at a desk counter that was mid-chest high and the ladies sat at their desks looking up.

"Are you familiar with the Caroline Pryce Walker Act?" Warren asked. "It was passed over for the 2009 budget and we're asking they take a very, very hard look at it this year. The reason we're here is because our daughter passed away on August 6th. She was 11 years old. We promised and I promised her as she laid on her bed for weeks before she died, I said we will do this somehow, some way. I will not let this lie," he told the women at their desks. "If the senator could get even a glimpse by looking at the DVD and reading the letter that we've addressed to the President which, by the way, we've been told has been hand delivered to Mr. Obama," Warren continued as he showed them the document. "Here's the DVD and the letter."

The women never got up from their seats.

The Browns walked out of that office and others who had refused to meet with them with a baffled look on their faces, but a stern resolve. People saying "no" did not intimidate them. Rather, it made them want to point out how ludicrous it was for them to turn their backs on a law that was passed without any opposition.

The next visit was friendlier ground and with a familiar face—Senator Sherrod Brown from Ohio.

"Good to see you, Sherrod," said Warren.

"Thank you. Nice to see you," the senator said, extending his hand out for a firm shake and looking down at the documents the Browns had with them.

"We got the letters hand-delivered to all the right places," the senator told them.

I jumped in after a few more pleasantries were exchanged.

"What's your initial reaction to having the Browns down here in D.C.?"

Sherrod was more than comfortable with us rolling our cameras in HIS office unlike others who did not want anything to do with us.

"The Browns are making a difference and this is why it's so important," said the raspy-voice senator in his first elected term.

"How can something like childhood cancer be overlooked by our representatives after they already approved the funding?" I asked.

"It takes someone like Wendy and Warren to really humanize it and say this is somebody we know, somebody close to us, this was our daughter, somebody in our neighborhood that this affects so dramatically," Sherrod told us.

"Senator, what types of things are you hearing from the Appropriations Committee?" I inquired.

"I'm talking to them. We just hit them from all different directions and get their attention," he answered.

"What could be more important than childhood cancer, children dying of cancer?" I asked.

"Nothing's more important. That's why I'm optimistic that we're going to get this help," he said. "Amazingly enough, there's never been the focus in our country, not just the government, but business, foundations, and states that have had the focus on children's illness the way that there should be," he opined.

He explained that there have been efforts in testing and research, but much more for adults than kids. "We've not put the effort into children that we should," he said.

I knew with that statement I had to ask about those other projects that do get the attention and the focus when sick kids are ignored.

"Can you describe for the folks in Northwest Ohio how some of these other things get funded like scenic trails and studies for oysters when the childhood cancer act doesn't get the attention?" I questioned.

"Well, there are..." Sherrod started saying and then stopped as if he was amazed himself how those kinds of things get the money they do. "That's a tough question," he continued with a look of contemplation now draped on his face. "There are a lot of needs...there are reasons that government spends money on things. It's hard to come up with a better reason than pediatric cancer...and that's why we're working on this so hard," he summed up.

It was a good meeting. He told the Browns his next step was to talk to Senator Tom Harkin from Iowa who was the Chairman of the Labor, Health and Human Services, Education Sub-committee of the Senate on Appropriations Committee. Sherrod was counting on Harkin and the conference to hear the importance of this money for our children.

Warren told us later in the day during one of our debriefing interviews that Senator Brown's commitment was amazing. "His level of compassion and passion for the issue I think is maybe even a little more intense than it was when we met him on our porch this past summer," he said. Sherrod had the Browns motivated even when other offices let them down.

Senator Arlen Spector from Pennsylvania let the Browns sit down with a staffer. Warren and Wendy did detect a level of inexperience in the young lady who sat with little to say during the discussion.

Senator Harry Reid from Nevada let a woman named Carolyn Gluck talk with the Browns. Warren and Wendy said Gluck was very positive but very truthful about how their request was not an easy thing to get done. She said Senator Reid was one of the main sponsors of the Caroline Pryce Walker Conquer Childhood Cancer Act. He was definitely for the release of the funding. They said Gluck told them it helps when people like the Browns make a personal visit. "She said it is good for representatives and senators to hear from people like us," Wendy revealed about the closed-door meeting.

The busy day continued with a walk to the Rayburn Building where Ohio Representative Marcy Kaptur's office was. I had known the representative for quite some time now and even covered the push she made to have the National World War II Memorial constructed. I was in D.C. for the dedication sending back reports via satellite. The idea for the WWII memorial came from a veteran in northwest Ohio. It was one of my first big stories to cover when I arrived in Toledo. This time my mission was much different. Instead of getting something done before more WWII veterans died, I was trying to get more funding before more CHILDREN died of cancer.

"Thank you very much for coming here," said Representative Kaptur as she greeted the Browns in her office. Our cameras were rolling. She did not care.

As they sat together in the long-time politician's office that was decorated with pictures and awards Kaptur had received and photos of the very area she represented, Shawn and I took a couple of chairs off to the side and listened in.

"There is a funding disparity, Representative Kaptur, where adult cancers get singular funding for each type of cancer and pediatric cancer just gets an overall budget," he said.

The Browns started talking about Alexa and her struggles. "She told one of our best friends that she was not afraid to die but she just didn't want to leave her loved ones," Warren revealed with more tears surfacing. "Whatever you can do to that (Carolyn Pryce Walker Conquer Childhood Cancer) Act to make it a reality in a funding nature, we would very much appreciate it," said Warren as the weight of the water was too much for his eyelashes to hold any longer.

Wendy stepped in and described how the Ohio Department of Health made the circle of study larger to include even more people from northwest Ohio. Warren told her there were a lot of people who wanted to blame ODH and the Ohio EPA but he wanted to focus on society and dumping that put so many harmful agents into the water, air, and soil. He also told her he was ultimately looking for a cure and not necessarily for an answer to the cancer cluster around his town.

"I can't understand what's taking that study so long," said the congresswoman.

Warren and Wendy talked about how it would have been even longer had it not been for me and WTOL getting involved and exposing the agencies' lack of commitment to extra testing and using all the resources they had promised.

"Every child's life is precious," she told us after the formal talks with the Browns had concluded. "It takes a lot of strength to do what (the Browns) are doing," she recognized. "We'll try to do what we can to help them achieve their goal. No family is immune from this. In fact, we know in our region of Ohio the cancer rates are much higher in all categories and we have to understand why," she said with the worried look of a protective mother.

Kaptur was a member of the House Committee on Appropriations. She said her next steps were to see what the "disposition of the committee" was for the funding. She needed to familiarize herself with budgets, and see what more the local schools like the University of Toledo Medical Center could do when it comes to research.

"To have this level of childhood cancer…should be an alarming crisis," said the congresswoman. "One where the alarm bell should go off and say we have to do more there. (The Browns) raised my awareness that the pediatric cancer area has not gotten the same level of funding which is really quite surprising," she concluded.

The Browns left Kaptur's office feeling a bit better about how the more recent part of the day had gone. After coming out of the gate so positively, then receiving mixed messages, it was good to hear some support from such a veteran on Capitol Hill.

Their next appointment was with Congressman Bob Latta who represented that same area where the cancer cluster was located. He had shown support for the Browns for quite some time as he worked behind the scenes fighting for money to be released.

"Hi, Bob," said Warren as the representative walked into his office. "Good to see you."

Bob was a shorter man in his early 50's with a thin build but a strong conviction when talking about spending priorities in D.C.

"When it comes to slicing the pie, certain voices are getting heard more and we have to make sure we're covering everybody," said Latta during his meeting with the Browns.

"Your efforts have not gone unnoticed and I appreciate it very, very much, Bob," said Warren as he sat across from the man who had just recently pushed for at least $10 million to be released. The request had not done much yet but there was hope.

As I talked with the congressman, I wanted to get a feel for his thoughts on how money is spent in Washington. I thought it would be interesting to get his perspective since he was a newcomer to the seat that was vacated by the sudden death of Paul Gilmor. Bob had only been serving as a House rep since 2007.

"There are billions of dollars, trillions of dollars being spent," he told us. "And you can say we are spending money on things we shouldn't be spending money on. We talk about what's in these bills and then look at the amount and it's just like why? Why are we spending money on this?" he continued. "They pass a bill in the House for $700 million dollars to take care of wild horses. $700 million! What's more important kids or horses? We're going to start focusing on the most important things…It's finding these cures that we got to have for these cancers," Latta said putting funding into some perspective.

It had been a long day and our last stop was to meet with people involved with CureSearch. That is an organization committed to pushing for more funding and research for pediatric cancer.

We went to one of the upper floors of a tall building where there were balconies overlooking the Capitol Building. The Browns had collected thousands of dollars through all kinds of fundraisers. We rolled tape on the presentation of the generous gift to Kate Shafer who was the Director of Advocacy at CureSearch.

"We want to present this to you…" said Wendy but could not even finish before Kate started hugging her and then Warren joined in. I guess I don't have to tell you that tears made another appearance during the donation that was full of real dollars, hard work, and memories of little Alexa.

The check was for $8,071.35. It seemed like such a smaller number when you compare it with $30 million a year for five years. But remember, none of that money from the Carolyn Pryce Walker Conquer Childhood Cancer Act had been released. So, since the government did not give an appropriated dime to pediatric cancer research, the Brown's check of eight grand amounted to more than the $150,000,000 that Congress passed and President Obama signed.

We wanted to pull Kate away from the emotion and ask her some questions about what this trip really meant to the people in Washington. We had a vested interest, so we knew the importance but as someone who saw their own lobbyists work on the congressmen every day, what was her view? We changed our location to the balcony so we could have the brightly lit Capitol Building as a backdrop for the interview.

"The Browns are really doing something for future generations of American families and children," said Kate without hesitation. "The thing that influences members of Congress more than anything else is that 'personal story' of why that issue is important to them. The power of two is unbelievable," she told us when there was a slight chill in the air but also a warm feeling of conviction surrounding this trip.

That night we all slept well after putting plenty of miles on our soles and much sharing of our souls.

Day two of our Hill walking tour included brief visits with the offices of Senator Daniel Inouye from Hawaii, Senator Thad Cochran from Mississippi, and Senator Tom Harkin from Iowa. Warren described the level of interest from the staffers ranged from "She assures us the bill will be addressed…it has to be addressed," to "he would take a hard look at this" to "she kind of evaded that whole area of childhood cancer and went into NIH and watching them and making sure what they research is important." Some of it was positive but we never really got the feeling that people understood the true sense of the urgency needed. It was slow, business-as-usual for our governmental machine.

The best part of the day, though, included a quick—but action-packed—discussion with Congressman Dennis Kucinich from Ohio. The Browns were from his state but not from the district he represented. He decided to meet with them anyway. He gave the Browns 10 minutes despite us calling ahead to set up a more involved interview.

Dennis was a tiny man who was very thin. He was a presidential candidate in prior years. His small stature never got in the way of his big dreams.

There was a long pause between when we arrived at his office and when he finally invited the Browns in. He needed "to get ready" said one of the media reps.

"What a tragedy to lose a beautiful child," Dennis said about the Browns situation. "Wendy and Warren make the case that we really have to have more attention paid to researching childhood cancer. I will be talking with people about the bill and see if there's a way we can move it along," he added.

"He's got a fiery personality and he said he is definitely going to address this bill," said Warren looking back on the quick visit.

"In the 10 minutes we were there, we couldn't have had 10 better minutes with anyone else," Wendy told us afterward.

At the end of the day, we were standing in the Hart Building where so many senators' offices surrounded us. During our final interview of the trip, I asked the Browns how they felt the past couple of days had been.

"I think we have effectively gotten our message out," Warren told us with a bit of a tired feeling in his voice…not a defeated sound, but more exhausted than anything else.

"The majority would like to and the majority even said they would look into the funding problems with the cancer act," said Wendy. "A few, of course, they didn't show interest, but overall, it was very positive," she concluded.

"I told Alexa I would not relent and if it doesn't happen this year, I won't relent and I will be back next year," Warren said even after the tiresome, hectic schedule.

When they got home, it was time for them to follow up on the meetings they had and get more people writing letters to help influence those who control the appropriations.

Shawn and I shot a few on-camera sequences where I stood in front of the camera and explained more aspects of this story. One shot started on the outside of the Capitol Building and panned down to me on the lawn. "One of the most interesting aspects of the governmental process here in Washington, D.C. is that members of Congress can pass all the bills they want into law, but if there's no funding…some of those bills are rendered meaningless," I said. As those words came out of my mouth, there was still hope in my head that the "meaningless" aspect of the governmental process would

NOT be the case with the Caroline Pryce Walker Act. But there's that word again…hope.

When I got back to Toledo, I knew there were so many angles to this story we had to tell. It would be all about the clear determination of the Browns, the people who welcomed their visit, those who did not, those who are picking up the fight; those who are leaving it to someone else; the memories of Alexa, and the next steps for the Browns. I also knew I had to shine a spotlight on what projects were getting the money when kids dying from cancer were left out.

The first night of my reports revealed the efforts of the Browns and their impressions of the Washington system. I also showed the way they were fighting, not only in their daughter's memory, but for the thousands of others getting knocked down or out by the cancer punches being thrown across the country.

The second night featured a different tone. I started the taped story with a soundbite from Warren about the overall goal of their trip. "Give it the $30 million dollars it was intended to have and give it for five years in which it was intended to be funded," he said talking about the Caroline Pryce Walker Conquer Childhood Cancer Act.

Then came my voice. "Even though the House and the Senate passed it without any objection from any members of Congress, the appropriations committees (which decide what gets funding) did not give any money in 2009 for that law. The National Cancer Institute does get federal appropriated funds for childhood cancer issues. In fact, in 2008 it received 192 million dollars overall for pediatric cancer. However, that's out of a total budget of 4.8 billion dollars NCI gets from the government. That's four percent of NCI's overall budget. The Caroline Pryce Walker Act would give 30 million dollars a year to help increase what cancer victims call 'a disparity in childhood cancer funding.' On their trip, the Browns emphasized this need to those on the appropriations committees," I explained.

"It was passed over for the 2009 budget and we're asking they take a very, very hard look at it this year," Warren said during one of our interviews.

I then told our viewers where some of the money was going. "News 11 found other earmarks that were funded in 2009 instead of kids with cancer. (Here's what the watchdog group, Taxpayers for Commonsense, has reported.) Senator Tom Harkin from Iowa helped appropriate Missouri River Fish Mitigation at $57.4 million, planning and design of the Edward M. Kennedy Institute at $5.8 million...that's not for the building itself, just the planning and design...and $1.8 million went to Swine Odor and Manure Management Research.

"Patty Murry...senator from Washington State sent us a statement saying she was a co-sponsor of the Caroline Pryce Walker Conquer Childhood Cancer Act. In 2009, she approved money for fish mitigation...$83.3 million, a Timber Fish Wildlife Program for $1.7 million, and a million dollars for potato research.

"Hawaii Senator Daniel Inouye...$8.8 million on a Historic Whaling and Trading Partners program, $750,000 for finfish research, and $469,000 for a Fruit Fly Facility.

"Thad Cochran, Senator from Mississippi...Performing Arts Activities...$6.8 million, a Fitness Center...$6.3 million, and something called 'Wood Utilization'...$4.5 million.

"Herb Kohl, Senator from Wisconsin...spent money for livestock identification, forest products lab equipment, and an Ice Age Scenic Trail got one million dollars before the Childhood Cancer Act got a dime.

"All of our requests to speak to the senators were denied when we were in Washington with the Browns," I told the viewers on tape.

"The House of Representatives' earmarks for 2009 are interesting as well," I continued. "A presidential library...$22 million, a chapel...$11.6 million...a commuter rail study, grape genetics, oyster recovery and more all received money last year and research for childhood cancer didn't get any appropriations," I pointed out.

I actually had to cut down the list of all of the interesting projects that got money. I did not have time to keep showing the point of just how much sick kids had been neglected for other "important" things.

I ended the story with a plea from the Browns. "More letters need to be written to Congress, to your senators, and to your representatives.

More phone calls. More emails supporting the Caroline Pryce Walk Act," said Warren, staring into the camera and into the hearts of anyone who bothered to listen.

Apparently, someone heard the message. Just a few days after our "projects" report aired, we had a new report to tell our viewers.

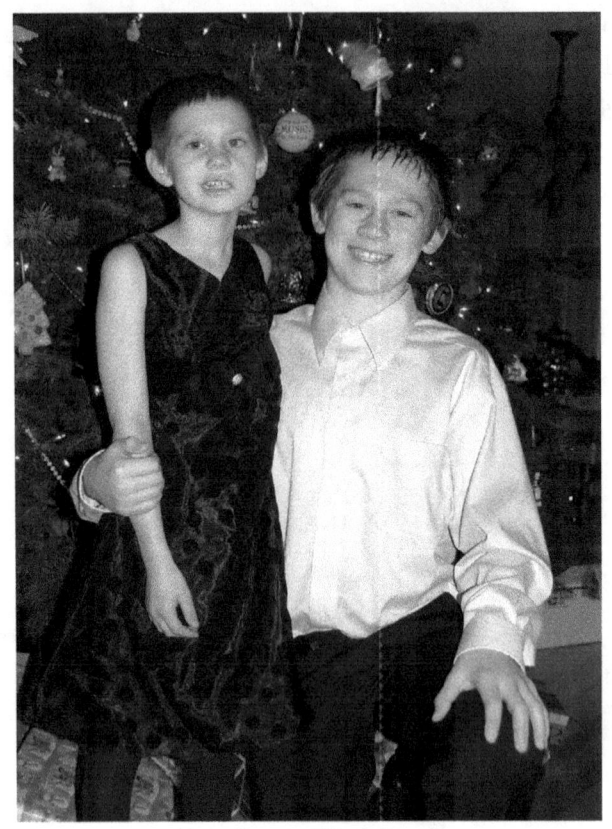

Alexa Brown, Ethan Brown

"I have never been, especially with the associated tumultuous commercialism, a Christmas holiday fan. Subsequently, I cannot express in words what an empty season this has become since Alexa has gone to Heaven. In the same vein, I cannot express what a heightened meaning this season has for me when I think of Alexa sitting at the feet of Jesus and hearing speak words of comfort and wisdom."

Warren
On CaringBridge.com

chapter 24

"New details tonight on the Eastern Sandusky County Childhood Cancer Cluster and the efforts to fund research," said our anchor, Jerry Anderson, on an early-December night. "Bowling Green Congressman Bob Latta tells News 11 he's asking for full funding of the Caroline Pryce Walker Conquer Childhood Cancer Act of 2008. Full funding of that bill is the primary goal of Warren and Wendy Brown, parents of the late Alexa Brown, who died earlier this year of cancer. 13 fellow Ohio lawmakers co-signed Latta's letter to the director of the Office of Management and Budget," Jerry informed our audience. Another ball was starting to roll.

The bright glare of media attention on how little attention childhood cancer put a lot of pressure on the agencies in charge of the study. The spotlight on the lack of progress more than likely created a sweat on the brows of the Ohio Department of Health and the Ohio EPA. My guess is the feds and top politicians were making more and more phone calls to the agencies. I soon got a phone call from Robert Jennings from ODH.

"Jonathan, we'd like to sit down with you and talk about what's going on with this study," said Jennings, who was one of the media relations reps for ODH.

"OK. When would you like to do that?" I asked while sitting in the news van on my beat-up cell phone.

"We'll be in Toledo on the 15th and we'd like to have your news director sit in on the interview," Jennings told me. It was an unusual request to have my boss there. She had never been with me before during our interviews. I had no problem with that. In fact, I kind of liked the idea of having my news director, Andi Roman, there to see what kind of impressions she got from Robert Indian.

"No, problem. We'll see you on the 15th at the station," I told him as I hung up the phone. I looked forward to the face-to-face sit-down. I had a feeling though, they were upset. They should be, but not because of my reporting. They should be upset with the way the state conducted this whole "investigation."

Both men arrived on time for the interview. I met them in the lobby. They were cordial enough with handshakes and a couple of smiles. I will say these guys probably were not bad people, but I think the Ohio Department of Health was just in way over its head on this massive mystery.

As we sat down in our dimly lit conference room with a large table built for 16 people, Andi and I were on one side. The "Roberts" were positioned on the other side.

Robert Indian started by going over the initial steps of the study from day one when he got the inquiries from the Sandusky Health Department. He told us the agency had several different initiatives including investigating "legacy sites" in Sandusky County. Those are places such as WWII dumping grounds, any areas with evidence of improper disposal, and the Davis Besse Nuclear Power Plant that was near the circle of study. They did questionnaires for the families and then followed up with new, more comprehensive questionnaires later after finding out more about the cancer cluster. They set up monitoring stations on rooftops looking for any possible contaminants. They did a survey of all the schools. The Ohio EPA did stream samples and soon they would be going into people's homes and measuring radiation levels.

As they gathered information, Robert Indian told us they noticed a surge in cancer cases in 2005 and 2006. "If there was something that came through the area then you might have had an impact on births," explained Indian. However, he went on to tell us the fetal deaths, low-birth weight rates, infant mortality, and birth defects turned up nothing. No glaring numbers popped up on his radar.

"So, based on that outcome, is it still transient in nature?" I asked.

"It may have been. We really don't know, but the environmental sampling to date has been negative," Indian pointed out.

Indian told us that we should not put "too great an emphasis on the circle" of study that it was "just a piece of the puzzle." However, he was the one who brought up the expanded area of focus during a meeting in May. I pointed to that meeting and how he talked about the need to look deeper than just the Clyde-Green Springs-Green Creek Township area.

"Those maps we presented the first time around…this is the first time we've ever done this. It's been a learning experience," he said with a straight face. I thought to myself…wow. This was the guy who was in charge. Someone who was saying to a reporter on tape that it was a "learning experience." I, too, was learning something, or at least confirming my suspicions. This study was in trouble. These families were in trouble.

I pointed out to Indian that along the way the number of children in the study ranged from 38 to 28 to 35. It had been all over the place. If we had a circle of focus, then why the variation?

"It has fluctuated, that's right," Indian said with a bit of vigor. "The mapping is not perfect and when you take a look at what's reasonable to include and what will enhance our probability of finding something, we want to go with this 35 number," he continued.

"Of those 35, have they all been contacted?" I interrupted.

"No. Some have moved away," he shot back. He said some of the only information that was reported to him was the patient's name and where they lived.

"So, of those who are still at the addresses listed?" I asked trailing my voice off.

"The letters are going out very soon," he told me as he leaned back and looked down. I got the feeling that he knew I would be surprised by that. I had just reported a month ago that the additional families in the past had not been contacted. Here we were a good month later and still no communication.

"We didn't want to do this piecemeal…having some people contacted today and others in two weeks," Indian tried to explain. "We know where some people are. We've talked to them on the telephone, but they have not received a letter yet," he added.

Indian went on to say when there was a new case to consider in the cluster study, ODH gets a name, age, birthdate, type of cancer, address of diagnosis and no contact information for the families.

"Would it help you if the way the cases are reported would be changed to include more information?" I asked, now leaning on the table with my arms stretched out to indicate a bigger amount.

"It could be helpful, particularly for childhood cancer because… hospitals aren't there to do this for the Ohio Department of Health. They're managing their cases. They're not into the public health initiatives. So, we would have to tinker with the reporting rules," he explained to us.

I immediately thought the entire system was broken. There were no true common grounds in this fight. I'm sure people do not want kids to get cancer, but, if what he was saying was true, then they sure were not working together to help figure out what was going on with pediatric cancer issues.

"Could people push for those changes?" I asked.

"That would be helpful," he said.

The immediate next steps were for ODH to finish a comprehensive survey with a more atmospheric angle to it. It was more detailed and ODH had worked with the Ohio EPA for help on what questions to ask.

"This is a new cancer risk-factor questionnaire that has been developed along this way and it does put a heavy emphasis on environmental issues," said Indian.

"So, based on this study, you've come up with a new standard?" I questioned.

"Yes," he said without hesitation.

So, here we were in a tiny room in Toledo, Ohio talking about groundbreaking ways the state was trying to tackle how to research these kinds of cases in the future. What are the procedures? What should the protocol be? Who should be involved and what steps should those agencies take? It was all being learned on the fly and

I was learning in this conference room what I had suspected for a while…this cluster was unlike any other the experts had seen. It was trailblazing in and of itself.

"We've got some ticking time bombs out there," said Indian, about what kind of environmental factors there could be in this first-of-its-kind childhood cancer study. "People threw car batteries, paint cans… if you could get it in your car then you could throw it in that hole in the ground…then we cover it up and said it's all taken care of. Well, it's not," Indian told us as the camera was rolling the entire time.

"We don't know what causes childhood cancer," admitted Indian.

It was a telling admission, but what followed was even more eye opening.

"Why don't we have that answer?" I asked, staring him straight in the eye.

"Well, people need to be more supportive…be very supportive of more money going into what causes cancer particularly in children and so the next generation of scientists who follow me when this happens, they will know what to look for," he said with a straight face and serious tone. "Right now, that's what makes this job tough. I just don't know what to look for," he said with a sigh, sinking back into the chair.

I, too, leaned back from my previous position of being hunched over the table. The room was silent. There was the problem. We had a person who was charged with the duty of finding out why our kids were dying and, at the very least, why they were contracting this terrible disease. This man did not even have a solid starting point. Yes, he was doing some of the investigating to rule things out, but the foundation of causes was in the molecular level. There were not enough pieces to put together to even form a foundation on this one. No one can stand to get a better view, so we were all swimming in confusion and this was the man who was telling the Ohio EPA what steps to take next. I thought to myself this was all rubble, broken rubble with no rhyme or reason to it all.

"Our focus is on quality and doing the job right and that's what we'll do," Indian told us as he wrapped up the hour-long interview.

He said the focus was on quality and doing the job right, but in the same breath, he said he did not know what he was looking for. How then did he know it was "quality" and "right"? He didn't.

We were now three plus years into this cluster situation and the families had gained no answers. However, they had gained some friends in their fight.

Just two days after our meeting with Robert Indian and Robert Jennings, when the harsh reality hit about how problematic the state's investigation really was, there was some big news developing. Really, really big news.

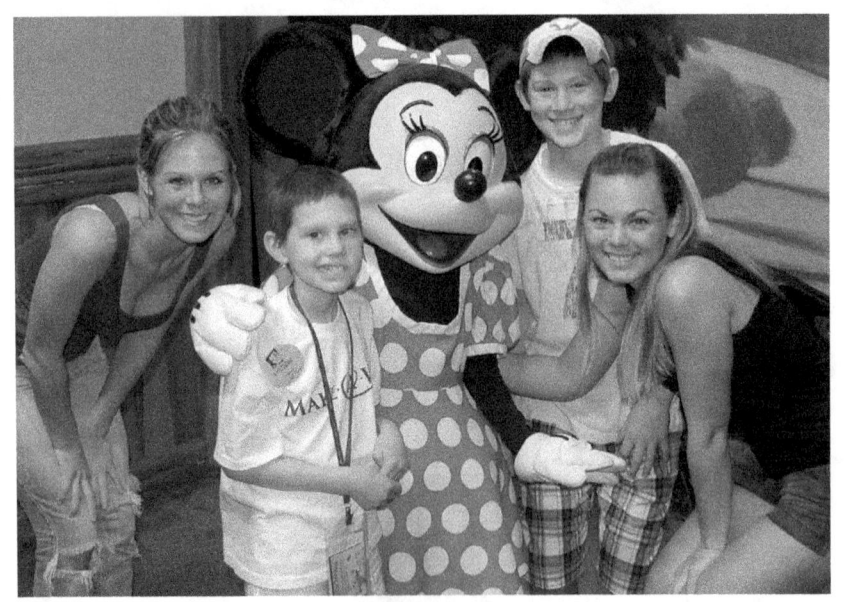

Abby Brown, Alexa Brown, Ethan Brown, Amanda Brown

"It's relationships! Forget money, prestige, perceived power, it is relationships that we mold through the forge that make the holidays, and any day—special! The word forge is intentionally used as sometimes making relationships work really needs to be the proverbial iron on the anvil! Alexa knew this with every fiber of her being her testimony to all of us it that we better be about the business of rally caring about each other rather than paying any attention to the matters in life that just don't matter!"

Warren
On CaringBridge.com

chapter 25

"Jonathan, call me. It's Warren. I have good news, my friend."

That was the voicemail I got after waking up on a cold mid-December morning. I knew that our reporting made it down through the channels of Washington, D.C. because the previous day I got a hand-written note on U.S. Senate stationary. It was from Senator Sherrod Brown.

"Jonathan, Very good work in Clyde on Thursday. You are making a real difference. That's what real journalism is all about. Sherrod."

It was an unexpected note but one that was very much appreciated.

"Hey, Warren. What's going on?" I asked after dialing his number.

"Jonathan, we did it. We got people to listen to us," said Warren. "They released some money. Now, it's not all that we had hoped for, but our efforts have not gone unnoticed," he continued with a slight cracking in his voice toward the end of that last sentence.

"Wow. Well, what happened?" I asked starting to smile on my end of the phone.

"Well, check your email. Kate Shafer (from CureSearch) just sent out some information. It's millions, Jonathan," he told me. "After you check it, then give me a call and I can sit down later today if you want an interview," he added. Wendy had gone to Georgia with a friend so Warren was all by himself.

"Okay. Great. I'll look at the email then talk to the station about getting down your way tonight. This all sounds good, Warren," I said hoping for a response because at this point it appeared to be positive but I did not know the details.

"It is good, Jonathan. Let's talk tonight," he said as we finished up the conversation.

I quickly ran upstairs to wash up and wake up a little more. I grabbed my laptop and it seemed like an eternity for my work email page to load. As I stared at the screen with the little icon spinning as the computer thought about the next step, I could not picture exactly what Warren was alluding to about the "good" news. What did he mean? Was it a lot of what we hoped? Would it make a difference in the overall fight? All of those questions raced through my mind until I was finally able to get logged in. I say "finally" but it was probably about a minute…maybe less than that. Either way, it was still too slow compared to my heart rate.

I got through the junk mail and the normal work emails about the day's news and there it was.

"Hard work resulted in an unprecedented additional $5.6 million in appropriations dedicated to childhood cancer. This is more money than has ever been specifically appropriated by Congress for childhood cancer," Kate wrote in black and white. My mind, though, was in the gray area.

It was great we were able to get money set aside. Unprecedented money. We got people to listen. We accomplished something. But it was only $5.6 million. The Pryce Walker Act called for $30 million. Did they not listen to Warren and Wendy? Did they still not get it? Why didn't they get it? What more could we have done?

It was all confusing. It was fantastic that we started the ball rolling, but it was nothing compared to what it should have been. It was a first-of-its-kind, but Congress was still spending millions more on a freaking fitness center. Good God! My head hurts.

That night Shawn and I made it down to Clyde and the Brown's home. Warren wore a hooded sweatshirt on and sat far into their couch. He was deep in thought. His shoulders were relaxed. I could tell the news had been playing on his mind just about as much as my brain was doing the good-bad gymnastics.

Warren had to call Wendy in Georgia. "I got just a little bit emotional," Warren explained about the phone call. "It's a small victory inside the battle and a smaller victory inside the war, but at least it's a victory," he added.

He was right. I knew it from the start, but it was hard not to think about all that other money. It was a victory.

"You've got to start somewhere," said Warren, who further explained that Kate Shafer told him the money would be used to develop a registry for pediatric cancer. It will help researchers, scientists, and doctors better understand the numbers and cases of childhood cancer and help them track down more information.

Warren went on to say that he thought the message of 40,000 people translated through Wendy, himself, and, of course, Alexa. "I told her we were going to do it…and we've done a part of it and because of her, we're going to do all of it," Warren told us as the camera was rolling.

He said that he and Wendy would go to D.C. as often as is necessary to let people know just how severely our children are suffering with this disease. He described the need for more attention on the aspects of life that really mattered and that when you considered our kids, presidential libraries were not that important. "Fish and horses and bricks and mortar…none of that stacks up to children who have really true life-threatening issues that have to be dealt with," he said, but then stopped and took a breath. He looked on either side of him. No one was there. He gave a half-smile and sunk deeper into the couch.

"What is it, Warren?" I asked acknowledging that he was clearly thinking about something.

"Jonathan, this was the spot," he said pointing to the couch cushion. "She read that story to you right here…'The Scariest Day of My Life'… and here we are three years later…" he said stopping again and shaking his head. It was starting to really hit him what had happened because of his promise and his and Wendy's efforts.

The tears started to flow…taking that familiar path again, but these tears had a different meaning on their well-known journey. There were at least some happy tears intermixed with the I-miss-you tears.

"I do believe that she is in Heaven surrounded by my mom and dad and Wendy's mom and dad and she's saying to them…'Look at your kids…look at what your kids are doing to remember me,'" he finished with a burst of tears now pouring out of his eyes.

I looked at Shawn. We stopped the tape.

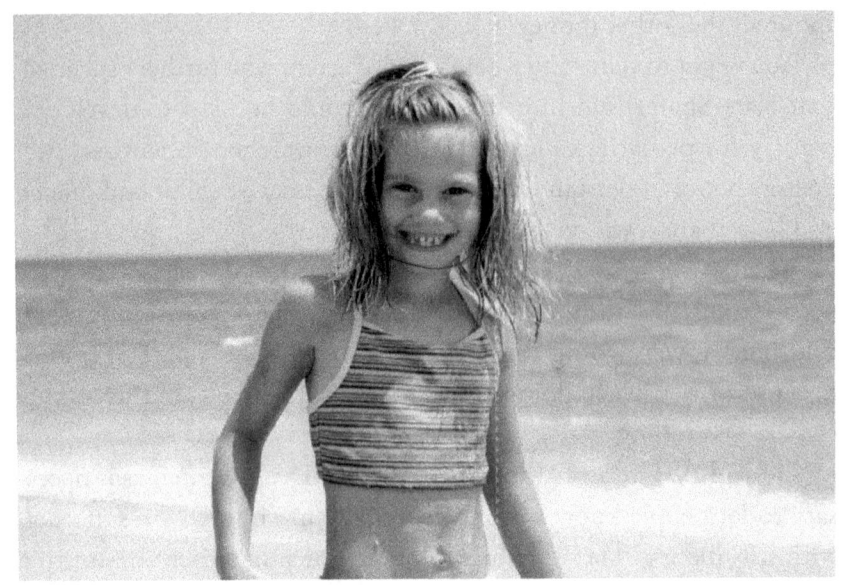

Alexa Brown before she had cancer

"Simple things reminded many of us of Alexa as we travelled down here. This morning as we ate breakfast at one of the hotels we've stayed in many times, Wendy started crying as she recalled Alexa heading straight for the Fruit Loops. Much will be different every time we travel to 'her beach.'"

Warren
On CaringBridge.com

chapter 26

"This is not the grief-stricken, cancer victim's father preaching," said Warren in a WTOL interview. "This is the common man for common sense," he added.

Everything about the governments' (local, state, and federal) approaches made Warren so upset, he decided it was time for him to take a shot at changing the system. In early 2010, Warren announced he was running for the U.S. Senate.

It was a seat that was about to be vacated by republican George Voinovich. However, Warren did not want to run with any particular party. He felt both Republicans and Democrats had lost focus on what really matters to real people. So, he decided to run as an independent.

Of course, one of his main issues he intended to fight for was childhood cancer research, but he was not going to be a one-trick pony. He had many ideas about budgets, taxes, and term-limits.

He had many people gathering signatures to get him on the ballot, but the problem when you run as an independent candidate is the system is against you. As an independent, you have to gather 5,000 signatures in Ohio in order to move on with your U.S. Senate candidacy. However, when you are a Republican or a Democratic candidate, you only need 1,000 signatures. Big difference.

By the way, at that time, if you wanted to be an independent House candidate, the number of signatures needed is based on voter turnout in that congressional district during the last general election for governor. That could add up to thousands and, at the very least, be so much more than the 50 signatures required for House candidates from the major parties.

With all of the obstacles, Warren's run for the senate was short-lived. At least he tried to do something with a political machine that he felt was broken and skewed to work only for those attached to the main political parties. Those in power make the rules, and they made the rules much more difficult for those not interested in only following party lines. The failed candidacy attempt did not mean the Browns were done with Washington, D.C.

Meanwhile, the state of Ohio continued the testing for possible problems that led to the cancer. This time radiation test strips were placed in some of the homes of the cancer victims.

"There's one right there," said Wendy as we walked around her house. "It kind of looks like a name badge."

Wendy showed us where the 11 "name badges" were placed. White strips in the kitchen, in the family room, in bedrooms were all trying to see if the Browns were exposed to extra amounts of radiation in their own home.

Wendy acknowledged it was not going to help Alexa and she was not really sure it was going to help anyone else. "They're doing the testing," she told us. "I don't think they're going to find anything, but you never know."

Warren was on the same page. "I think it's worthwhile checking," he said with a smirk. "Whether or not it comes to a conclusion, I have my doubts," he continued with a shake of his bald head.

The Hisey family agreed to put up the tags as well.

"There's one on the wall," Dave Hisey explained as he pointed to the test strip. "There's one in the bedroom and it seems they are spaced apart to cover many of the areas of their house. We don't have any answers yet and where are the answers going to come from? I don't know," he said with a baffled look on his face.

Dave then explained to me that Tanner was on a bit of a roller coaster with his treatments. Some days were good like when Tanner was able to play baseball, but then the ugly head of cancer would throw Tanner a curveball of its own. "You lose faith that investigators are going to find anything because it seems like everywhere you look there's nothing to find," the discouraged father revealed. "It sure seems like there's a reason out there somewhere."

And there was no seeming about it. The overall roller coaster of this health nightmare never stopped. At that point, who knew how many more families were standing in the cancer cluster turnstiles and they didn't even know it.

During all of the testing, lobbying Congress, and running for the Senate, there was never a pause in the effort to keep doing what was right in preserving Alexa's spirit on earth. The Browns found time to organize the first-ever Alexa Brown Memorial Golf Outing. The money raised would be given to a scholarship fund that the family established. It was for a student of what would have been Alexa's high school graduating class. It was one of two non-profit ventures. The other was Alexa's Butterflies of Hope which accepted donations to help all the cancer cluster families with various expenses related to taking care of their children.

Sleepy Hollow Golf Course in Clyde was the site. It was a nice setting for 18 holes with a challenging layout for extreme amateurs of the game like myself. As we approached the course, we noticed about a dozen teams with their clubs on the back of their carts.

"Thanks for attending, everybody," said Warren on the bullhorn near the modest clubhouse. He knew it was their first attempt at a golf tournament. He was just happy any amount of money would be collected to help the cause.

"There's not a minute that I don't think about Alexa and I miss her so, so, so, so much," said Amanda Brown while wearing an Alexa shirt from a previous fundraiser. It was hard for her to ever talk about her little sister without tears welling up.

"I wish we really didn't have to do this," said Amanda's older sister, Abby. "I wish it wasn't a memorial, but it's nice to remember Alexa and to see the community come out."

Tanner Hisey was there. So was his sister, Tyler Smith. It was often the case that other members of this cancer cluster showed up and supported the focus family of whatever the event happened to be.

Seeing the faces of those surviving the disease and those who have no blood ties to the victims really showed just how much genuine care and love there was in Clyde.

"I'd like to...oh...you're going to make me cry," said Wendy during a moment between getting the golfers out and organizing the last-minute details. She took a second to reflect. "I'd like to thank everybody for coming, remembering Alexa, and helping her name to live on," said the mom who had cried more than any mother should have to.

"I know she's watching down right now on us," Abby added with a lean and a hug for her mom.

After the outing, the Browns' target went from the golfing greens to a different kind of green—money in Washington D.C....again. Warren and Wendy attended a national event for pediatric cancer research called "Reach the Day." It was sponsored by CureSearch and is held every year. People from across the country gathered in our nation's capital to meet with dozens of congressional leaders and to urge them to dedicate more funds.

Warren and Wendy took a handheld camera and taped the new experience. "It's all done to help us reach the day when every child with cancer can be guaranteed a cure," said Wendy. "Until that happens, our work isn't done."

As they stood with 250 others on the Capitol steps, in politicians' offices, and around the power of D.C., the funding goal wasn't the only thing on their minds. "What I did find myself doing was reliving Alexa's experiences," admitted Wendy.

"There's a vacuum in my soul that will never ever be filled again," said Warren on the same note.

During the event, there were seminars on new experimental treatments. "It's really promising therapy, but without research dollars, it stops with experimenting on mice," said Wendy in a this-is-our-reality tone.

Even more reality would set in about three weeks after the D.C. trip. It was time to return Alexa to "Her Beach."

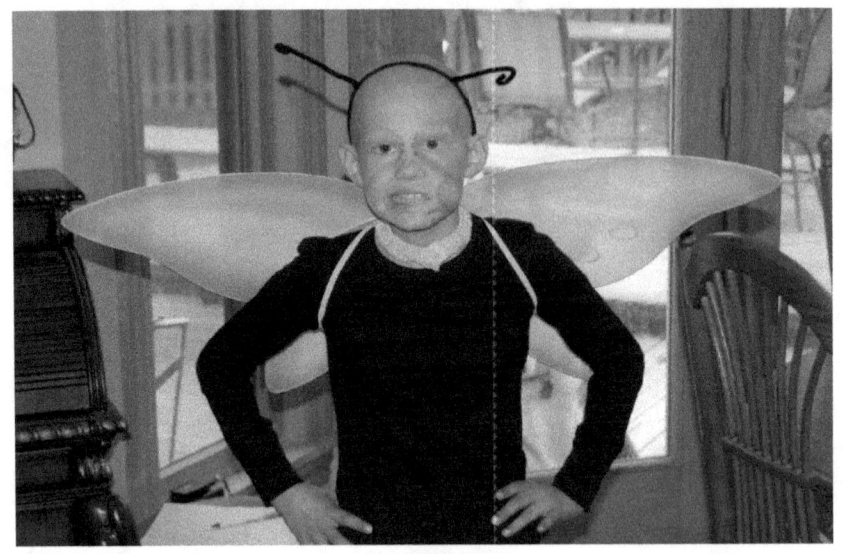

Alexa Brown

"Butterflies were meant to fly. Your wings await you after you've shown so many how to fight on no matter what. You and your family are so strong. You are amazing."

-Alisa

chapter 27

I called Warren before the family was about to leave. "Are you ready to do this?" I asked.

"I don't know, Jonathan, but it's something we have to do for her," replied the worn-out father. "Thanks for calling. We'll see you soon," he said as he hung up the phone.

"This is Alexa's room and today we leave for her most favorite place in the world," said a tearful Warren Brown who was taping on a handheld camera. You could hear him crying as he narrated the scene in his baby girl's room.

"That's Alexa's suitcase from last year. The suitcase has stayed there exactly the way she packed it," he said emotionally. Alexa had been planning to get back to the Outer Banks in North Carolina before she took a turn for the worse. She would never make that last family vacation."

I love you, Alexa, and I miss you, honey," said Warren now with obvious tears and more than a quiver in his voice.

The emotions were raw the whole way down south. The family rode in separate cars. At a rest stop, Warren tried to get a few words on tape with his children about how they felt heading to North Carolina without Alexa for the first time.

"Hey, buddy, step over here for a minute," Warren told Alexa's brother Ethan. Warren had the camera rolling outside their SUV and Ethan wanted nothing to do with it. He walked in the opposite direction of his father. "Nobody really wants to be making this trip without Alexa," Warren continued on tape.

My photographer, Shawn, and I left for the Outer Banks about a day after the Browns took off. The drive took us all over the place where our GPS included crazy back roads in West Virginia. We laughed at some of the small towns like Paw Paw where the redundant name became a running joke throughout our trip.

There were school bus stops along a highway that not only had speed limits of 60 miles per hour, but neither I nor Shawn ever saw a house anywhere near the bus stops. How do kids climb on a bus there? We chuckled to pass the time, but we knew once we got to North Carolina there would be more serious and emotional work to handle.

As we made our way through Virginia, the family was settling in with a big picture of Alexa by their side. It was the 4th of July.

"Alexa loved fireworks," said her mom, Wendy. "She loved the noise of fireworks. She just liked everything about them," she added.

We arrived in North Carolina and drove toward the house in South Nags Head. I couldn't help but notice rows and rows of oceanfront property, sand, and license plates from all kinds of states dotting the cars parked in driveways. I also couldn't help but notice how many families were walking around, biking, or taking a dip in the ocean. At one point, I saw a little girl about Alexa's age when she passed. She actually had a purple suit on and purple towel slug around her neck. Purple was Alexa's favorite color.

We pulled up to the house. It was just before sunset. It was a large, 6-7-bedroom home specifically meant for big families and/or multiple families to enjoy the ocean. The Browns saved us a room. That way we were with the family and could document this dramatic physical conclusion of Alexa's Journey. There was a big fireworks display planned at some nearby sand dunes.

We drove with the family to catch a spot with the thousands of other vacationers who were at the Outer Banks for very different reasons.

"Alexa needed to be right underneath the fireworks where the little pieces of ash would come down," Warren joked, but his laugh was short. "This morning as I was looking at the ocean, I realized once again how this place will never be the same for us. It is absolutely never going to be the same." Just like the family will never be the same without Alexa.

"It was two in the morning on the Fourth of July last year when Alexa woke up and said, 'Mommy, my arm hurts' and that was when she had a stroke," Wendy recalled. "It's kind of what I think about, unfortunately, when I think about the 4th of July."

The next day we woke up before sunrise. Shawn was known for sleeping in, but he was definitely ready for this shoot. He was up before I was. His camera was in hand and he was already getting shots. The beach was about 50 yards away from the back of the home.

I wandered from the house to the beach where Shawn was set up. I noticed the horizon had signs of the sun ready to make its appearance. It was a nice purple sky. I smiled.

As Shawn shot video, out of the corner of my eye I saw Warren making his way to the water. He was shirtless with long swim shorts. He held a long fishing rod in his hand. He wanted to snag fish and soak in the sunrise.

As Warren flung the lure, we waded through the water for an interview.

"It's a great day to come down and throw a line in the water...try to catch something," said Warren. He, too, noticed the fantastic sky with the sun peeking through. "It's almost like there's nothing wrong in the world when you look at that. You bank those few moments in your mind when you feel like there's nothing wrong in the world."

We asked about what this trip meant to him and what he expected from the experience. "I know there are going to be a lot of tears shed that will be sent back into the ocean as the waves roll in," he told us while looking at the endless vision of water.

"Why show the world your pain, Warren?" I asked, referencing the family allowing us to follow them to North Carolina. There was a pause.

"We sense a real responsibility to keep the message out there and let people know that pediatric cancer is not going to go away," he answered. "This easily could be your family. I don't wish that on anybody, but everybody needs to know that this disease is so very real. This story is repeated 13,000 times a year. 13,000 times a year a child develops cancer. Right now, every day two classrooms of children will develop cancer. 4,000 other children who have developed cancer will…," Warren paused to gather himself for a second before continuing. "Will end up with Alexa in Heaven. That's why we're doing this. Until Congress does what it allowed itself to do and funds childhood cancer research to the tune that Congress has funded other disease issues, this story will not end."

Later that day, we followed Warren to a nearby souvenir store that had been a must-visit location any time the family was in town.

"Alexa just loved to get something as a reminder of 'Her Beach,'" Warren told us as he walked among the T-shirts, mugs, and beaded jewelry. "It didn't have to be the most expensive thing, but always had to have that something special to evoke the memories of great times," he added as he choked up.

We left the store and headed back to the house. By that time, Alexa's sisters had made their way to the water. We took our camera down to join them.

"I look out here and I don't see a little kid playing in the sand," said Alexa's sister, Abby. She was sitting in the sun on a beach chair. "I don't see a little girl excited to see dolphins, but I know if she was here, that's what she would want. There's a huge part of my heart that isn't here," she added.

"Does it get any easier as time goes by?" I asked.

"I guess, but there are so many times I just don't know what to say about the grieving because it hurts so much," Abby told us in a very frank tone. "It's a deep pain that just doesn't go away."

"Why are you willing to share your story with us and everyone who will see this story?" I inquired.

"Until it hits your own family, I don't think many people realize how serious it is. We saw it firsthand and I hope someday that other families will never have to go through that," she answered.

As Abby finished her last statement, Amanda walked up to towel herself off.

"I think a lot of families take for granted the health of their kids," Amanda, Alexa's other sister, told us. "If it was me who had gotten sick and had cancer, I would have been okay with that because I'm

23 years-old. I've lived a long enough life. There are kids who are two, and four and eight and 11 like Alexa and who don't live to be a teenager. They don't get to grow up and go to the prom and get married and have kids of their own," she added.

Ethan joined the conversation. "We just have to spread the awareness about childhood cancer so more people know what to look for, how to prevent it, how to fight it, and how to take a stand for more research," the young man said, sounding years beyond his age. "Those in charge of making decisions about funding and research really need to look inside themselves. See what's actually important. They need to take care of the next generation. They need to stop worrying about all those other things that they are giving senseless money to. They need to focus on what's really important," he told us.

By this time, Wendy had set up her chair to join the family on the sand. "You can live the rest of your life and try to ignore childhood cancer, or you can do something about it to try and make it better for somebody else," she said, staring out into the lapping waters tickling the sands near her bare feet. "As I sit here, I think about the past three years and all the treatments Alexa went through and all the things that were so hurtful to her. Those things don't need to happen to any child. We need to concentrate on making things better. We'll keep on fighting forever," she added.

Alexa's cousin, Ray Brown, also made the trip to be with the family during the emotional time. "Alexa's battle is over, but ours has just begun," Ray said. "Until they find a cure we need to keep plugging away. Anyone who wants to raise awareness for cancer research is a friend. The world needs as many friends in this fight as possible."

Abby's fiancé, Greg Reynolds, added to that note. "Everybody sees the success with breast cancer awareness, so why not childhood cancer?" he asked.

As I wrapped up the interviews for the day, I knew the sole reason we were in Nags Head was about to happen that evening. The family was going to spread Alexa's ashes. That's where she wanted to be.

"The thought of having to spread my child's ashes across the beach is quite frankly really overwhelming, Jonathan," said Warren, who once again could not help but get emotional. The family planned the ceremony to mark their tribute to Alexa.

Shawn and I wanted to be on the beach before the others so we could get shots of them making their way to the water. As Shawn got into place, Warren came out of the house with his purple shirt on. He had a shovel over his shoulder. His head was down as he walked toward the water. He did not pay attention to us. I wondered what was going through his mind. I also wondered why he had a shovel. We soon found out.

Warren scoped out a spacious area so that everyone could participate. He then took the shovel and wrote Alexa's name in the sand. When he was done, he stepped back. He looked for a second. He then put the shovel back in the sand. He made a huge heart around his daughter's name.

Just as he finished, the family walked single-file through the sand and to the newly formed heart. They all wore some clothing with the color purple in it. Ethan was hugging Alexa's large, framed picture. He carried it to the ceremony.

Alexa was there. After all it was "Her Beach."

Earth to earth. Ashes to ashes. Dust to dust.

epilogue

I recently wrote the Ohio Department of Health asking about the childhood cancer cases. Here's the response I received:

"The final report from the Ohio Department of Health (ODH) on Childhood Cancer in Eastern Sandusky County was released on May 26, 2011. This report summarizes multiple analyses that were conducted and presents the results of interviews with cases who were willing to participate. ODH is not actively investigating a childhood cancer cluster in the area, but uses data from the Ohio Cancer Incidence Surveillance System (OCISS) to monitor the cancer burden in the state of Ohio. A county profile for Sandusky County was released in 2019… According to the May 2011 report, 'there was a total of 35 known children with verified cancer among residents 19 years and younger in the eastern Sandusky County cluster area diagnosed during the years 1996-2010'…ODH is not actively investigating a cancer cluster in Eastern Sandusky County at this time. If concerns are raised, ODH will work with Sandusky County Public Health."

There were areas of soil found to be contaminated, but the study claims "…there were no exposures or variables that were common to the 21 (of the 35) children with cancer who participated in this profile."

In the same Discussion and Conclusion section of the study it states "…to date there has been limited success in identifying the cause of childhood cancer."

To which I say, it's obvious the "limited success" is because not enough is being done. That's why I wrote about these families. That's why every single profit I make from this book will go back into fighting this devasting diagnosis.

You are the next voice we need to carry this message to those who can do something about pediatric cancer. Write your representatives. Communicate with research hospitals and organizations about the need. Demand better from our public health leaders. Just be the voice for those little ones and their families.

There is no greater love than that of a parent for his or her child. When that child hurts, the pain strikes our hearts, but our love should never waiver.

We need to love our children whether they are our own, in our extended family, or the neighbor down the street. Protect them as if they were the only ones in the next generation.

If we can't do that, then why are we here? Why exist if just for our existence? Love extends beyond our boundaries; imaginary or real.

The children most in need bring the most out of all of us. Bring your love to them in every way. A hug, a donation, a law. All are significant in securing their peace and our responsibility.

more from the CaringBridge.com journaling

I haven't shared many emotions or feelings lately, just ways to help. Tonight, I just feel like sharing a little bit of my heart. My friend had a baby girl today. She had her at St. V's (Alexa's hospital). Walking around the hospital tonight was just horrible. The hospital holds no good memoires for us. Brain surgery, chemo, radiation, MRIs, etc. (as well as being the place where my grandma was 6 years ago after her massive stroke). But what hurts the most was walking by Alexa's gift shop. The gift shop was one of Alexa's favorite places to shop. I could hardly even look in the door. These are the times when I have to believe and know that she is so much better now. She is not in pain and perhaps even visiting a much better gift shop in Heaven. I'm still selfish, I want her here.

Abby
On CaringBridge.com

Sleep is not coming tonight in any semblance of the word. It is hard to lie in the bed where Alexa was present only a few days ago. Everyone is composed most of the time but the little things set us off. Going to Walmart (Alexa's favorite shopping venue), riding on the bike trail (Alexa loved riding her bike), finding one of her lists (Alexa was the ultimate list maker). Preparations for her Celebration of Life Service are underway. The girls a preparing a video for the preservice.

My brother, Frank, will be presiding. Friends are helping with many other matters surrounding the service. Thanks for keeping us in your prayers.

Warren
On CaringBridge.com

Four years—sometimes it seems unreal that Alexa has been in Heaven that long. She'd be getting geared up for her sophomore year in high school in the next week or two.

She is so missed by her family that words can't describe it.

Thanks for the years of moral support and prayers for my family.

Blessings to all,

Warren
On CaringBridge.com

about the author

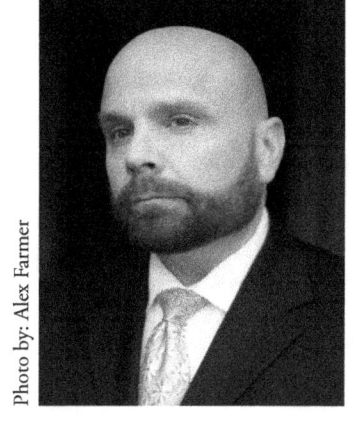

Photo by: Alex Farmer

Jonathan Walsh has been an investigative journalist for the past 20 years working for television stations in Texas, Pennsylvania, Minnesota, and Ohio. He's earned 8 Edward R. Murrow Awards including a national Murrow for his storytelling. He's won 13 Emmys and 18 Associated Press Awards including several for Best Reporter, Best Investigative Reporter, Best Enterprise Reporting, Continuing Coverage, and more. He currently works for the E.W. Scripps station News 5, WEWS in Cleveland, OH. He loves and adores his wife Alisa, and two children Kalib and Lizzie. He's motived and inspired by the families he's covered. He knows you will be, too.

CPSIA information can be obtained
at www.ICGtesting.com
Printed in the USA
FSHW011333180820
73059FS